The Ancestral Now

The Intersection Between Deep Time, Primal Movement, Nutrition, Magic and Ancestral Consciousness

RAMON CASTELLANOS

The Ancestral Now: The Intersection Between Deep Time, Primal Movement, Nutrition, Magic and Ancestral Consciousness - Written By Ramon Castellanos

Published by Ancestral Dragon Scrolls

Theancestralnow.com

Cover by Ramon Francisco Castellanos and Crystal Marie Castellanos

ISBN: 979-8-218-05262-1

First Printing: 2022
Printed in United States of America

ON GRATITUDE

There are many to whom I feel immense gratitude, for, without their aid this book would not be possible.

Firstly, I would like to thank The Ancestors themselves. Thanks for the wisdom, inheritance and blessings they offer us individually and as a collective. At times, this book poured through me and I could literally feel The Ancestors reaching through time, quickening me into its writing. This book is, at least in part, a treatise and devotional act to them. And in this vein, I thank my grandmother, who is now an ancestor, for being my first magic teacher and fostering my creativity.

I want to thank my wife for her ongoing support, patience, love, encouragement and belief in me. I would like to thank her for her incredible heart and bright spirit. Not to mention, for editing this book! She inspires me daily, and without her ongoing gift of presence this book may never have come to fruition.

I would like to thank my mother for giving birth to me, for through her, the ancestral lines transmitted their intelligence to me. She acted as a portal into this domain, and so without her, this book would not exist. Her continued support and love for me aid in connecting to the deeper ancestral stream in ways that foster blessings.

I thank my father, for through him, the ancestral line on my paternal side reached through time and aided in the creation of my inheritance from the ancestors. His drive, tenacity and persistence, although expressed very differently in me, are an inheritance that has allowed me the necessary disposition to pursue some of the experiences that shaped this work.

I would like to thank my mentor, the wide-ranging Mushtaq Ali Al Ansari. He is someone who has been very giving with his time and energy to me, even when it was difficult. Years of conversation with him about wildness, human adulthood, hunter-gatherers, "human superpowers", and his overall shaping influence, prepared me for this work. Though, I add that this writing occurred in my interpretation, so inadequacies in the work are mine and are not reflective of his influence.

I would like to thank my magic teacher and incredible and generous human being, Fabeku Fatunmise. What I learned from him, in regards to magic and The Ancestors, has forever changed me. This book would not be possible without his influence, at least not in its current iteration. What I learned from him has been instrumental in writing the section on "Ancestral Consciousness". Though, I add that this writing occurred in my interpretation, so inadequacies in the work are mine, and are not reflective of his influence.

I would like to thank the wolves and wolfdogs at Wild Spirit Wolf Sanctuary that were major teachers to me in regards to what being a wild animal means. Especially Flurry, Forest, Quinn, Leia, and Naia. Flurry and Forest have passed on, and may their spirit be blessed.

I would like to thank my good friend, Dr. Craig Wells, D.O. His teachings, influence and depth of scope on energetics, alchemy, Osteopathy and alignment with destiny, have been life changing and set me on a clear path that led to this book as a possibility. The healing work he has done for me has further accommodated this work as a possibility.

I would like to offer a deep, heartfelt thanks to Mohammad Fahad Abrar. A lifelong friend whose support has made it possible for me to stay in the

AT THE GATES

CHAPTER 1

How to Navigate the Forest of Ancestral Forces

"*We truly are a species with amnesia. We have forgotten a very important part of our story.*" - Graham Hancock

There is a desire to reconnect and rediscover parts of ourselves that we can feel are calling out from our depths. They call us with a yearning for something that is not so clear to many. This is a book about context and our alignment with that context: a set of conditions that emerge from a strong connection to the ancestral forces that have shaped us over billions of years. This text explores elements of this ancestral molding and what they might mean for us as both citizens of the earth and children of the modern space age.

This book is also centered around the digestion of our past, the deep primal experiences rippling through time. Digestion in many ways is a type of discernment. We must be able to tease apart the nutrients from the poisons, extracting and receiving the nourishing, and eliminating the waste. A massive transition in the human story occurred with our move away from hunter-gatherer tribal cultures into contemporary urban and suburban life. This life we lead now is a roaring fire fueled by agriculture and it has left much of our innate humanity, our species-level inheritance, undigested and unprocessed. We have become sick because of it.

For some, if not many of us, modernity has carved out and butchered parts of our wholeness. It is no wonder many of us feel disconnected, disorientated, and deflated in ways that carry an existential sense of loss. This ache often goes beyond a clearly defined storyline that is identifiable in our own lives. It is possible that this pain is really a type of thirst; a yearning for the nectar that is an awakening of our primal and ancestral consciousness. To this end, let us do the work of attuning to the primal and ancestral forces for the sake of our wholeness, a deeper sense of aliveness, and a root system that allows us to weather the storms of society.

The strength, power and support of our ancestral core is reaching forward from the past and surrounding us with open arms. To embrace these potent forces we must be willing to do the difficult but rewarding work of unweaving the spells woven and etched into our souls. On the other side of this is a more meaningful life: more vitality, improvements in health, a deeper sense of belonging in the world, less fear, and more love. The ancestral is not a panacea but it is the only remedy for some of our embedded wounds.

While it is true that there are many layers which may feed into the sense of having lost an essential wholeness, the ancestral is a critical part of who we are. It is enmeshed into the fabric of our consciousness at such fundamental levels that it could be said we swim in an ocean of ancestral currents buffeted by waves of deep time. It is my hope that the perspectives and exercises laid out in this book help to deepen your relationship to these prevalent forces within you, wherever you are in your relationship with them.

Here, the ancestral can be related much to true, wild territory - with some difficult terrain to navigate. We may find some obscuring density, creatures that go bump in the night, and elemental forces of unspeakable beauty as well. It is possible to get lost and there are some dangers that may be lurking in the shadows. So, I hope to offer some tools, skills, and a map of sorts that can go a long way towards helping us navigate the ancestral safely. The journey is worth it. At the heart of this wild place is home.

The Areas of Focus

What can be related to as "ancestral" is vast, and a book about ancestry can cover a lot of ground. For the sake of putting this resource to practical use, we need some degree of focus. The topics we will cover have entire volumes written about them, so I openly admit that the treatment of each topic is by no means exhaustive. This is as much out of sheer necessity as it is by design. The true value of this *Ancestral Now* concept is to experience how a few key lifeways can dance together with modern life. The real magic is in how all the ingredients support, blend, and meld into one another. We are not serving up a delicate caviar here; we are cooking up a nourishing stew.

The primary areas we will explore are:

1. **A broader more inclusive look at ancestry that goes beyond our individual family lines and even extends beyond**

humans. This will tie us into the archetypal ancestors and place them into relationship with the long history of life on this planet and beyond. From this look into our ancestry, we will draw a few useful practices relevant to being a 21st century Homo sapiens.

2. **We will touch upon our relationship to movement.** This will open the door to primal and ancestral movement forms, and how we might play and dance with these ideas in our own life.

3. **We will chew on the human condition through the lens of food** with ancestral nutrition, and how one might go about being a modern hunter-gatherer.

4. **Finally, we saunter into the smoky and shadowy domain of animism, ancestral veneration, and our relationship with the dead.**

All these areas of exploration are, broadly speaking, largely accessible to the majority of humans in these modern times, regardless of whether you live in a concrete jungle or you find yourself in an actual jungle. Whenever I have discussed a relationship to ancestry, accessibility has always been important to me. The overwhelming majority of our ancestors lived wild lives, enmeshed within the elemental world that springs forth from unobstructed, direct contact with nature. In many of the circles that explore ancestry with this realization in mind, a tendency towards "wildness", "primitive human skills" and "ways of life more closely aligned with tribal cultures" is often pursued. There is a lot of merit in this, yet we do not necessarily need to leave our contemporary lives behind, move into the wild, begin weaving baskets and hunting elk to connect with our ancestry. It is possible to do this if you choose to, of course.

I have lived a certain version of "living in the wild." I spent ten years living in the high desert wilderness of New Mexico, where I called the Zuni mountains home. I did so as a senior staff member at Wild Spirit Wolf Sanctuary, a facility located at least two and a half hours away from a major city. I have experienced what it is like to live in small, minimal and bare housing made from large logs. Not the quaint log cabins or tiny houses that are popular today, but six-sided, traditional log cabins called Hogans which are little more than walls, a roof, and a dirt or concrete floor. For years I chopped wood and brought fire to life if I wanted to be warm. My wife and I did not have our own bathroom the whole ten years we were there and we "did as bears do" out in the woods if not in an outhouse. The elements had their way with me more times than I can count; I got caught in blizzards, got lost in the woods, got drenched in monsoons, slipped and fell in knee deep mud. I threw myself against nature out of utter necessity. I had close encounters with wolves, rattle snakes, bears, coyotes, bats, skunks, toads, hawks, and other wild birds. Some of these wild creatures I even had the privilege of befriending.

From my own experience, there is much reward, beauty, and aliveness that can come from the experiences of living a wild life. It can also bring steep prices to pay and many challenges to overcome which can leave one permanently altered in ways that are not always auspicious. This book is not suggesting that you live this way. In fact, this tome finds its magic in adopting practices and perspectives that can be readily accessed. If taken as a whole, they might, with the upfront cost of honest engagement, give you a clearer context for what it means to be a human.

Ancestral Now may aid you in cultivating greater degrees of wholeness. This happens in large part through the recognition that much of who we are in the present *is* ancestral. So much more than most of us realize has not been consciously chosen *by us*. From the vantage point of cause and effect, who we are today is the result of trillions of causes, conditions and their effects colliding, culminating, and reverberating through time. The whole of the evolutionary process from amoebas to fish, from reptiles to mammals, is stored within you. A series of memories, transformations, and transmutations held within the record of deep time reside in your cells.

From an archetypal level of what it even means to be human, the entirety of the human story is also present in your experience. All the hominids, tribal peoples, and paleolithic developments are at some level *a part of* you. This inherited memory is so vast that a singular unitary cell that is offered by each parent during reproduction leads to the creation of a whole human being. The embryonic process itself holds all the stages of evolution within it! You may have the nose, eyes, skin texture, hair, and/or proportions of an ancestor that lived thousands of years ago. Consider that many of your instinctual drives are shared by all humans and many creatures on this planet.

We are also influenced by many of the stories, traumas, and behavior patterns that have passed through time. Much of this has not been chosen by you. It is circumstantial. It is ancestral. Through the practices and trajectory outlined in this book, it may be possible to recapture more of our wholeness by reawakening our ancestral self.

Inhabiting a Personal Mythology

"Myth is much more important and true than history. History is just journalism and you know how reliable that is."
~ Joseph Campbell

I would like to encourage you to try and relate to the work in this book as mythology. There is magic in the ways we relate to the ancestral, and no degree of scientific study will ever reveal the mysteries contained in reclaiming our unique inheritance. I made that mistake in my early days exploring this whole arena of experience, chasing the reductionist dream. For this reason, I have left out citations on purpose. If something moves you, I encourage you to carve out the time for that exploration on your own. I do my best not to make claims that are not easy to verify with a simple internet search, that are not based on my personal experience, or that are not obvious once pointed out. In some cases, we will delve into topics completely outside the scope of modern western science.

While there will be exercises and strong suggestions laid out in this work, it is important to understand that as we dive deeper into the ancestral, we also discover more about who *we* are, both as individuals and at a species-wide level. This is the whole point. It may not seem like it at first glance, but I do not make a case for a "natural state" that we must try to recreate, enact, or aspire to. I hold that there is no such state. There are, however, intrinsic characteristics that we can discover. This is why the work in this is mythological, because it is real in ways that can only be experienced directly. How we engage with and embody the ancestral is nonlinear. We are literally shaped by these forces and I will lay out much clearer examples of what I mean by that as the book progresses. I lay out landmarks and principles of travel, but ultimately this relies on your immersion. I cannot hand you cookie cutter solutions. Your very body is the nature of the ancestors, and what seeks to emerge from it will take you further than any exercise. The key to understanding this is that the ancestral is already *here*. We do not need to *build it* so much as discover it *is* present and breathing. Then we just have to walk it out, fall down, get back up and keep going in the true resilient spirit of the ancients.

Nor is this done for nostalgia, or to create a type of "fetish" of our ancestors. We are seeking the inherent. In some cases, we may need to regenerate and regrow parts of ourselves that have been lost, dropped like a lizard letting go of its own tail, but the design is still inside you. With some effort, nourishing food, and rest, your human nature has you covered. The purpose of this material is to help you to organically awaken a sense of being more actively human, and present with the challenges and opportunities of the 21st century. This is about being *Ancestral Now.*

The Ocean of The Ancestors

"A river never forgets its source" - Yoruba proverb

It is a short-sighted, perceptual act to relate to ancestry exclusively through the narrow lens of our personal, genetic configuration and lineage, especially if our reference point is only a few hundred years. The reality is we have access to a much larger, richer, powerful, and deeper ancestral current - the ancestry of the human species itself. This stretches back through deep time, moving beyond humanity. It travels back through the tree of evolution, and finds its roots in the primeval oceans. Considering certain theories that contend life may have been seeded off planet, traveling here through space on crash-landed objects, ancestry may even extend *beyond* the ancient oceans. The broader human ancestry is akin to a river all of humanity stands within - subject to the pulls, pushes, spirals, and waves moving within it. Our own ancestry is much like a smaller tributary extending from this strong body of water. Life on this planet is the sea that creates the river.

When we refer to ancestry, there are different time frames and stages of development to consider. We could relate to any move: from amoebas to fish, to reptiles to land bearing creatures, to the first hominids then neanderthal influences, then Paleolithic hunter-gatherer ancestors and finally, early neolithic peoples. Where is ancestry in any of these cases? In essence, it is *all* of it. Unless referred to otherwise when referring to ancestry, I invite you to consider the bigger bodies of water that are "The" ancestors, more so than "our" ancestors. Of course, there will be a place for this more personal current as well.

Orienting to "The" ancestors is important for a few reasons. The first being that it opens us up and out of a fearful, jaded attitude that can understandably manifest if we are connecting purely to recent ancestry. Many people I have spoken to about ancestry have the immediate reaction that "My ancestors were terrible people." or some variation thereof. Ancestry is the very current of life that started wiggling about eons ago. These early life forms became sacks of ocean water that then began to walk on land. Through many winding paths, early humanoids emerged which led to our entire hunter-gatherer bloodlines. This represents *tens of thousands* of generations of tribal cultures. There is no statement about recent ancestry, even stretching back two thousand years, that can encompass it.

The last few thousand years of human history are not fully representative of humanity in the least. This time frame represents a drop of water in a very large bucket of evolution. Our recent, personal ancestry has had to contend with a world very different from the one our species evolved within. They found themselves outside their natural condition and were forced to break off pieces of themselves to fit. Looked at from a broad enough vantage point with compassion, decisions made may make more sense. That is not to justify atrocious behavior, but the last few millennia for humans have been akin to trapping wild animals in cages and expecting them to perform circus tricks. Those who relegate ancestry to a *few* previous generations are looking at the tip of an iceberg without recognizing the behemoth that is underneath.

I hesitate to make claims about specific time frames of how long humans in their current form have been on the planet. Credible sources refer to time frames anywhere between 250,000 to 2,000,000 years. Science, by its very nature, is always updating and while there are contexts in which working with these numbers are helpful, I am not so sure it is helpful here; this is not a work of science.

Another reason to approach ancestry in this way is that it loosens the grip of excessive cultural conservatism, where and when it is an unhealthy act. Culture can offer incredible gifts, as well as all-consuming traps. But this work is not about holding onto the past so much as it is absorbing it and aligning with it. If you do not understand the deeper stories that have led you here, you cannot integrate them into your totality.

The third reason is one of practical utility. Many of the greater gifts of ancestor work are found in the larger currents and not in the smaller ones. That is not to say that smaller currents do not have value, but I find they have less to do with major life trajectories in most cases. Consider that ancestral movement patterns, ancestral nutrition, the human heritage of magical practice, fundamental ancestral worldviews, deeper connections to the natural world, our resilience, and our innate ways of relating to one another all emerge from the large ancestral currents. Like any flowing body of water, there is momentum driving in a particular direction. In fact, so much of who we *think* we are as distinct individuals, is our ancestral conditioning taking place and exerting *its* influence. Some of this is specific to your recent line and some of it is deeply ancient. The desire for social interaction, warmth, food, movement, meaning, acceptance, and sex, to name a few, are drives you think you possess, but they actually possess you. You see ways to leverage objects, ideas, thoughts or attitudes because like all humans, you are a tool user. This extends the way our five senses are calibrated to how we orient in reality on nearly every level.

It is closer to the truth to recognize that there are personal and transpersonal currents to ancestry. The larger currents give rise to the smaller ones. Our own personal currents provide a ground that is necessary to explore, but I invite you to want to move deeper through space-time and reach into the broader, archetypal, ancestral forces that shape life on this planet and humanity itself.

SETTING THE STAGE IN STONE

CHAPTER 2

Our Hunter-gatherer Heritage

For the sake of clarity and expanding on the ancestral mythos in relatively stable ways, we will gently narrow our focus on the lifeways of tribal hunter-gatherers. This brings us to the doorstep of indigenous cultures that were and are living in the ancient way. We will also travel back through time into known elements of our Paleolithic ancestors that lived in the stone age, or the transitional space where hunting and gathering was still a central way of life - even if some agriculture was already taking place. In other words, we will explore pre-industrial humans in our lens of focus. We will do so because many of the practical applications of life-shaping ancestor work requires us to. We are still stone age hunter-gatherers in many ways, albeit we have nervous systems and other adaptations relevant to the contemporary world. While we may have fish and reptiles in our ancestry, we cannot really live like them in practical ways. We are human after all and owning the way in which wild humans live is how we weave this web of ancestral magic.

I want to set the stage and work with stone-age humans as a pillar for many of the major practices in this book. Please try your best not to be scientific or literal about adopting these changes if you choose to, as the purpose of this section is not to give an exhaustive scientific overview of how these people lived.

In the following section, you will find feats of human capacity, stories, general qualities, and lifeways that, for me, shed light on the magnificence of being human. These inheritances are a big part of what I relate to when I invoke the ancestors. When compared to the last few thousand years of the story we call "civilization", they provide a wondrous contrast to our potential and more true human nature. This is storytime in the spirit of calling in the largest possible human lineage in a relatively short section of this book. I will mix in elements from different timeframes and many cultures in order to express a generalized understanding of what *may* be inherent as a species.

Of course, this is by no means complete! I am just scratching the surface and being selective in order to offer context for the rest of the book and for those not actively engaged in studying indigenous and tribal cultures. If you are familiar with a lot of what I will share, please bear with me.

Storytime

To paint with broad strokes, it is not a stretch to say that our hunter-gatherer ancestors were incredibly skilled and capable. For the most part, their capacities far exceeded those of the general population alive today. They were vital and robust creatures, who by and large, were healthier and happier than most of us now.

The levels and types of stress they faced were vastly different. In many ways, their stress was more acute and short-lived, whereas our stress is chronic and pervasive. They also worked much less than we do and had more leisure time. They often filled their leisure time with lounging, playing music, crafts, social interaction, sex, and ritual. They ate better diets that were the epitome of fresh, local, organic, and in season. They lived in more rich and rewarding environments - not cubicles and asphalt. Their sexuality was, likely, less repressed than ours is today and they carried it with more ease. They experienced less trauma and more aliveness, and methods for healing spiritual wounds were built into their society.

If modern indigenous cultures are at all representative - and we have strong reason to think they are - ancient peoples had rich spiritual lives as well, finding deep meaning in the natural world and life shared with their people. Meaning and purpose were the water they swam in. There is a pervasive myth that floats around claiming they lived short, brutal lives that ended at age 35. It is clear at this point that hunter-gatherers can, and do, easily and regularly make it into their 50's, 60's, and even 70's. In general, they age in better health than many of their more "civilized" counterparts. However, they did have much higher rates of infant mortality. The statistical normalization of median lifespans that included infant mortality data is where the idea they only lived to be 35 years old came from.

Hunter-gatherers lived in close-knit communities. Tribes were, and still are, in many ways like large extended families. It appears that the hunter-gatherer tribes we evolved within could range anywhere from a few dozen to about 150 humans. In a world like this, your people and the lands you roam together with are your universe. The cosmology of your people is your cosmology. The health and state of the group are of paramount importance. These tribes lived and breathed community. As a result, tribal and indigenous cultures have family structures that function healthily, in contrast to the near-ubiquitous dysfunctional family dynamics most of us experience today in western culture.

Another misunderstanding that has emerged is that they were in constant competition with one another; impulsively stuck in survival of the fittest dynamics with each other. This is a projection of our own culture and studies from other species of primates onto our past. There is very little room for intense power struggles in such small groups that depend on one another for nearly everything. Imagine, if you will, living your entire life with the same 50 people; perhaps never even seeing another band of humans. These people would have either had a hand in raising you or grown-up side by side with you. You all would have spent decades eating the same meals, supporting one another in difficult times, praying together, dancing at the same fires, and hearing the same stories from the same elders as one. You have shared in the joys and pains of being human, and all you know is *this*. Now imagine that the group runs into lean times and many of the members of the tribe are unsuccessful with their hunts; but a few lucky, or very skilled, hunters bring home fresh kills. Does it really make any sense that those few would willfully withhold from the rest, feeding only his "chosen few"?

The notion that you would allow your loved ones to starve in the name of greed or status as the norm of the human story is deeply misguided and not indicative of how these ancient tribal cultures lived. Your own hoard means very little in a world where individual people own very little and most everything is shared. In many cases, paternal lineage is not even known. Tribes *are* the people. In a world like this, you simply *belong*. You feel a deep sense of having a place and a right to exist. Consider this in contrast to the deep loneliness and existential angst that is so ubiquitous in our cultures today.

The physical prowess of our hunter-gatherer ancestors was most impressive. A typical hunter-gatherer was quite fit with a high degree of physical capacity, much like any other wild animal. They were able to traverse varied, and at times hostile, environments carrying everything they owned. They did so as cooperative and cohesive units or had the ability to do so on their own. They had all the skills and adaptability needed to survive in unknown and unpredictable circumstances with no modern infrastructure to rely on. Some of them traversed ice bridges at the edge of the world and crossed continents without the luxury of high tech gear, global positioning systems, or prepackaged food rations. They navigated by looking at the stars, physical landmarks, remembering stories, using their intuition, and at times, by watching the behavior of other animals. With their natural abilities they were able to navigate through some of the toughest environments on earth.

When it comes to their athleticism, their qualities were just as impressive. There are documented stories of extreme endurance in existing tribal cultures. The Tarahumara of Mexico are able to run a few hundred miles at the drop of a hat with no warm-up, preamble, sports drinks, or supplements. This is to be expected for one of the top predators on the planet!

There is a form of hunting, which has all but died out today, that is still practiced by people in the Kalahari desert. It is called persistence hunting and it's like running a marathon to catch prey. It involves a group of humans continuously chasing after an ungulate for four to five hours during the hottest part of the day. The animal is then taken down after it has reached sheer exhaustion. Untrained people have tried persistence hunting and have failed because it requires the skill set of repeatedly locating and then separating an individual animal out from its herd. The learned skills have to be continuously utilized as the animal's higher speed allows them to get away, resulting in the need to be re-tracked, over and over again, until the animal reaches its exhaustion point. One of my mentors, Mushtaq Al Ali Ansari, a long time barefoot runner, likes to say "Endurance is one of our super powers." In fact, we are one of the best endurance runners on the planet. Our ability to sweat and consciously control our rhythm of breathing allows us to run for 24-hours straight if we wanted or needed to. We are the only animals capable of such a feat!

We have access to footage of Inuit tribes in northern Alaska that captures hunters as they launch themselves from boats like Olympic pole vaulters; except they are holding large harpoons, and landing on whales in freezing temperatures. Members of the Bajau tribe can hold their breath for 13 minutes at a time and walk on the ocean floor, as if they are taking a relaxed stroll, to spear fish. The Hadza people in Africa run through the dense and dangerous jungle floor barefoot to tango with, kill, and eat baboons.

Hunter-gatherer senses are so sensitive and alive that when observed by outsiders, many appear to harbor a sixth sense due to how finely tuned into the environment they can be. I recall reading a story about Australian Aboriginals who could, as a coordinated group, sneak into a body of water where a type of water fowl was present, hold their breath and progressively pull unsuspecting individuals from their flocks underwater. Ideally, the plucking of the individuals from the flock occurs without alerting the rest. They would then swim back out, carrying their kills in hand and in stealth. These same Aboriginals could throw spears, with the help of an object called a throwing stick, over 75 yards and hit a rabbit on the move.

Our gathering abilities were also quite substantial. The degree of knowledge held by tribes about the surrounding plants and their culinary or medicinal uses is astounding. The Yanomami of the Amazon routinely utilize around 500 species of plants for building materials, food, and medicines. Not only are they able to catalog the practical uses of hundreds of plants, they are able to distinguish poisons from nutrition without modern tools. One of their methods of determining this is by observing how other animals that eat the plant fare on it by watching its scat and general health. They then wonder just how similar or different that animal is from us to gauge potential crossover. If it appears safe on that level, they might take a small amount of its juice and place it on the skin, then lips and then tongue to gauge its effects. Does it sting, bite, or inflame upon contact? Then they may slowly increase dosages in safe and measured increments before it might be considered safe to eat. Plants are utilized to create rope, art, baskets, soap and complex tapestries requiring impressive fine motor skills and patience. It's essential to not only learn how to work with the plants but how to identify them, process them for a particular purpose, and put them to use in a multitude of ways. These are not skills relegated to a few members within the tribe, but are often common knowledge among all the people.

In general, hunter-gatherers have a lot of "free" time. It seems the amount of work required to sustain their needs ranges from three to five hours a day, and peaks at about 15-20 hours a week. Marshall Sahlins, author of the book, "Stone Age Economics", goes so far as to characterize them as "the original affluent society". In his work, he reports that the hunter-gatherers he studied shunned farming as "too much work". Of course, there are periods of want during certain seasonal changes, or when efforts did not yield favorable results, but to many hunter-gatherers, dying of hunger is inconceivable. On a whole, it seems that wild humans follow patterns evident in other large predators: short periods of difficult work with longer periods of lounging and rest.

Hunter-gatherer tribes also seem much better off from a level of sexual health when held up to modern cultures. They do not appear to have the same degree of sexual repression that civilized societies do, nor do they experience the degree of sexual diseases or violence we see. It would be inaccurate to say there is a standard all tribal cultures adhere to because sexual customs among the worlds many tribes appear as diverse as they are.

We find quite a bit of sexual diversity spread throughout the world of tribal cultures: polyamorous, polygamy, polyandry, partner-swapping, orgies, longterm pair-bonded marriages, same sex partnerships, and even sharing partners with people who visit the tribes. There also appears to be use of sexual magical practices where the sexual energy of many participants is brought together to heal disease, bring prosperous hunts, or bountiful yields. With that said, human sexuality does appear to always have some form of regulation, as customs, rituals and taboos do seem to spring up around sexuality; it is likely a feature of how we mate. There is a lot that could be said about sex, but we will leave it at the obvious truth that the modern standards we have in western society promoting a "mono replica relationship of one partner for life, preferably of a heterosexual nature," does not appear to hold from a tribal perspective. Combine all the diversity with the commonality of social nudity, close knit quarters, and less religious shame to contend with, and we have a much more *free* way of life.

Hunter-gatherers often appear to possess rich, spiritual lives based on animism (or what we in the West problematically call shamanism), a deep abiding connection to nature, and a devotional relationship to the flourishing of their tribe. Tribal cultures recognize that they belong to a multitude of ecosystems that includes the natural world of the elements; the realms of ghosts, ghouls and gods; the ancestral cycle of their people, and the domain of other species of animals. To hunter-gatherer tribes, the whole world is alive and vibrating with the breath of an ineffable spirit. They tend to develop a large array of rituals and prayers tied to life events, places of power, natural occurrences, and even practical magic where the goal is altering the flow of change. This is still quite common in much of the world and these types of magical and devotional ways of living emerge in almost every human culture. The one glaring exception are western "enlightenment" based philosophies that are deeply materialistic and reductionist, and rule western society.

Humans engage with the unseen realms by default; it is just a matter of how our consciousness is crafted. We seek meaning and purpose because we evolved in a setting where we would normally have it. We seek union with the divine because we always have. There is much more I could say, but hopefully this provides a foundation for much of what else will be touched on as we travel together through this book.

In general, we could say, our ancestors were robust, capable, spiritually alive, full of meaning, securely bonded within their communities, in tune with their environments, and sexually open. During their free time they would play games, engage in arts and crafts, dance, have sex, and commune with spirits and nature. They lived very differently, and in many ways, better lives than the ones most of us do today.

A Bleeding Wound in the Human Story

I shared what I consider to be some of the beauty, power, and gifts from our ancestral core. Those stories, capacities, and accomplishments inspire me and ignite a powerful fire in my soul. They impel me to aspire to move beyond the mediocre, for our heritage is anything but. However, we have to acknowledge that the pathways that lead from our tribal hunter-gatherer heritage to the modern world, are marred in stories of pain, wounding, and confusion. Much of the human story of the last 5,000 to 10,000 years is riddled with scar tissue, and the flow of nutrients from time and space before recorded history is restricted.

In many cases, it is a repeating theme in ancestral healing work to move around, above, or below the ancestors of the last few thousand years to find those who are avatars of the line before them - spirits who are representative of the last time the line was fully healthy and luminous. It is no surprise that this would be the case. The last few millennia have been rife with religious prosecution, sexual repression and violence, large scale war, genocide, slavery, disease, and a progressing weakening of our species. All of this, along with deep ecological damage on scales unknown to previous ancestral lines. It is this gap that has led to our current state of indigestion. Some cultures are more bloated and sick than others, depending on how far removed healthy ancestral inheritance is.

The real challenge is our tendency to look out upon the recent landscape and make assumptions about human nature based on that. Much of our actual humanity is shrouded under layers of thick, poisonous horror stories, that in truth, tell of time in the zoo of civilization, not of who we are by nature. In the words of Mushtaq Al Ali Ansari:

> *"Civilization can, in my estimation, be best modeled as a rather unique sort of zoo. Wild humans have been captured, taken from their natural habitat, and installed in fake habitats that superficially resemble their natural milieu. These humans are then taught tricks, and rewarded for doing the trick, while being punished for failing to do the trick. If you know anything about zoos, you know that this kind of captivity will quite literally drive the animals insane. Humans have developed coping mechanisms that keep full on psychotic break more or less at bay, so that they can be unsane rather than insane. They are religion, politics, and addiction."*

We are less human now than we were in the past, because captivity has twisted and warped our natural instincts and ways of life. This zoo is what we call a civilized society, and in many ways, its current organization is not your friend. The state of affairs of the last few thousand years is not representative of our organic humanity; it is an avatar of our prison. This is not necessarily condemnation of building civilizations; it is a recognition that the one we have built is not really in line with what makes our species beautiful and wondrous. The recent past has been akin to being darted and then waking up surrounded by walls, rules, and impositions meant to control our minds and strip us of our wildness. Yes, that world of our hunter-gatherer ancestors was not perfect. Of course there were times of difficulty, theft, loss, pain, war, and hunger. However, these traits were not likely the pervasive characteristics of our species for much of our time on this planet the way they are now.

An element of the conditioning that has taken place during "the fall" is that of a pervasive pessimism where we live in a world that is characterized by entropy and discord. It is this way, because we cannot see anything else; it has become our dominant mythos. We have no conception as a society of a world that could be different. Not a world without problems, but a world that is not *defined* by problems. The institutions of power that have arisen feed into the nefarious, color the lens of our sight, and reinforce these stories. So deep is this wound in our story that we do not know we are bleeding. Even many of the anthropologists who study our ancestors are subject to it. Look for this in the baseline assumptions related to our current "superiority" over the people of the past, and the materialistic worldviews that seep into their discoveries. The general theme is one in which we have evolved beyond their "simple, superstitious nonsense". So long as we hold this divisive, arrogant attitude, we will remain trapped. To continue with the words of Mushtaq:

> *"Now here's the most hilarious part of the situation. There is no zoo anymore. There is no zookeeper, nor is there any staff to maintain the zoo. We do all the work of keeping ourselves confined and conditioned*

> *to our captivity ourselves. We self condition for this and we condition all our offspring as well. We are our own captors. Escaping from the zoo is as easy as taking one step, but it's a step in a direction that you have been conditioned not to see. There is also the problem of being noticed by the captives. Part of the conditioning we all receive is to destroy anyone who notices that the zoo has no walls."*

The world is changing and it is more possible now for some of us to escape the zoo. There is so much distraction and degrees of constraint on the awareness of the mass population that many may not notice if you leave. The doors are wide open. The trick is this: you can set the parameters of what defines escape. You get to choose what being free means to you. We can do it alone, but the spirits of our ancestors are whispering their support and are willing to show us a part of the way if we put an ear to the ground and listen. The earth is vibrating with their bones, and if we pay attention, we can feel them rumbling.

CHAPTER 3

Hungry for Life

The Explicit Nature of the Ancestral World

The primal world, the very birthing ground of our species, radiates a reality that stands in stark contrast to the industrialized and civilized societies we find ourselves in. The ancestral world is deeply explicit. It is raw and pulsating with an immense vividness that inspires the senses and animates our aliveness on a consistent basis. We are starved for it; hungry and in desperate need of knowing ourselves through the natural world that birthed us.

We are blood.
We are bones.
We are guts.
We are oceans.
We are dirt.
We are sky.
We are wind.
We are thunder.
We are ecstatic shaking.

We are trees.
We are deserts.
We are spirits.
We are rhythmic music.
We are sex.
We are touch.
We are impact.
We are pulsating.
We are physicality.
We are rapture.
We are psychedelic.
We feast and famine.

These elements infused the lives of our ancestors for much of human history. We were alive and in the proverbial muck - a deeply rich and dense muck that helped shape the human mind, emotions, body, and soul. Ways of reconnecting to these elemental experiences can be inherently healing. Wild places and liberating experiences are where we can begin our escape. Places where we can release what is innate and already seeking expression. We find ourselves in those spaces because deep down we are human animals wanting to live like humans.

To be more "homegrown", as I like to say, seek out ways of having more enlivened experiences whenever you can. Be in nature, listen to the wind, walk barefoot outside, go into wild bodies of water, spend time in the mountains, drum, rattle, alter consciousness with weird plants (in relative safety), have sex with abandon and even with multiple people if you choose to, laugh with loved ones, paint your body with symbols, perform ritual and ceremony, commune with wild spirits, engage your consciousnesses with natural forces, talk to the dead, dance, eat rich and nourishing food, train your body into deep aliveness, and learn to simply be in silence. Be as human as you can be.

So much of modern life is dreary and dull. There is so little to enliven the senses and so much that drowns them out. It is a slow death without this form of nourishment. Dying of stagnation, our light extinguishes. Regaining a full capacity to *feel* is so critical. We need to be shaken and excited, because many of us are in a bondage of stasis. We need to be squeezed like a sponge so that the stress and strain in our systems can be released. Only then, can we actually experience true quiet - true rest.

The Cycles of Intensity

Many exist in the medium, never really feeling contrast. The medium is the rhythm of the mono culture, which breathes in a shallow, ho-hum, manner. Stepping into a deeper breath with a more full contrast begins to awaken the songs of our wildness. This gives us back the edge. Not the edges of better performance, but the sharpness of a blade that is in use. It makes us dangerous. Like many large predators, humans need to cycle periods of rest and intense activity. Finding rhythms that suit our innate nature is the way of harmony with natural forces and in aligning with the pulse of nature. In studying apex predators, we see regular cycles of what are called power-laws being expressed: a distribution of activity moving from no to low intensity, to moderate, to high intensity peak activities, that then move back to no or low intensity states. This is a basic wave form. Finding variations of this wave in our own world is a recipe for continuous aliveness. Doing so will help us break out of the hamster wheel and factory production-based rhythms that still perpetuate much of modernity.

For example, the more stressed and in need of healing a person is, the more that their healing ratio of cycling will need to be skewed towards rest and just being, rather than doing *more*. However, simply doing away with intensity for this person is not the answer. Intensity squeezes the sponges that are our nervous and endocrine systems. Humans are not single-speed creatures, and therefore, I recommend we find ways to shift gears on a consistent basis in a manner suited to our relative needs and constitution. This can apply as much to physical training routines as well as to other areas of one's life.

I will provide some examples of the different cycles of intensity below. I hope they inspire you, but you are encouraged to find ways to apply these degrees of intensity in a manner most coherent for you. It is of the utmost importance to keep in mind that intensity is a relative matter - your speed and capacity for mileage may vary at different times in your life. Some activities may require varying degrees of consistency, while others may require longer periods of rest from engaging in them. The following examples are generic and may, or may not, be true for you. The real magic is in the cycling of diversity. For me, intensity is about the stuff that gets you to let go and release into satisfaction. Intensity recalibrates us. The different cycles of intensity are as follows:

No Intensity: Creating consistent, predictable, easy-going routines for work. Reading. Being truly present with a cup of tea. Lounging around without the use of electronics. Deep pauses in awareness. Creating clay sculptures. Sky gazing and watching the clouds go by. Relaxing, hot showers, or hot baths. Sitting outside on the grass, feeling the earth, and feeling the wind. Sunbathing. Cuddling with and feeling the warmth of a lover. Gentle, devotional communion at an ancestral shrine. Going for a leisurely stroll outside. Easy mobility exercises to release tension. Sitting in trees.

Low Intensity: Going for short hikes. Contrast showers, shifting from hot to cold multiple times. Toning or chanting mantras. Snorkeling. A nice, overnight camp. Giving and receiving massages. Deep, but not difficult, physical training. Light eroticism with a partner and/or self pleasuring of some form. More engaged magical work than simple communion at a shrine. Deep immersion in playing an instrument. Being naked in nature. Passionate artwork.

Moderate Intensity: Joining drumming circles. Group singing. Moderate intensity dancing. Longer hikes. Basic free diving. Trail running. Slow to moderately paced sex. Easy parkour. Climbing trees. The moderate use of mind-altering substances like alcohol or marijuana. Strength training. Going out in the cold with minimal clothing. Depth jumping into wild bodies of water.

High Intensity: Using psychedelics. Intense sex with one or more partners. Peak experiences in nature such as rock climbing, surfing, or serious mountain biking. Intense, high impact exercise (relative to you). Full immersion in festivals like Burning Man. Ecstatic Dance. Serious ritual or magical work that deeply shifts your inner being. Endurance events.

Harvesting Pauses

"Music is the space between the notes."
- French composer, Claude Debussy

I first learned about the inherent quality of rhythm from one of my teachers, an extremely gifted magician, Fabeku Fatunmise. From his teachings I began to understand how different cultures, people, spirits, ancestor practices, and experiences all have their own unique, dynamic, and ongoing rhythms. Rhythms flow throughout our whole life, into our relations and our chosen trajectories, and we have consistent pulses that imbue the quality of our lived experience.

One of the hallmarks of modern culture is that it has a fast-paced, consistent, frenetic rhythm interwoven into it. We are always "on the go", constantly bombarded with low-grade energies, and constantly feeling as if "we must do this or that." The notes of this rhythm play one after the other with very little space in between them. Even when we have opportunities to do very little, we seek to fill the space with *something* and we flood the song of our lives with too much sound. Taking a look at the natural world and the animals within it, we see that this is not the case. Pauses and breaks in between activities consistently and organically occur. Animals just stop, breathe, sense, and feel their lived experience. They look around and take in their environment with a relaxed, open awareness. *This* is the space in between the notes.

If we take into consideration the world our ancestors evolved within, we can clearly see that they were not overstimulated the same way we are today. We can also see that living indigenous cultures generally swim within a slower current. Most hunter-gatherers only work a few hours a day and spend plenty of time in the quiet, easy rhythm of nature. Many of the great wisdom traditions also espouse the power and benefits of silence or pauses.

In today's society, our nervous systems are over-stimulated and it dramatically reduces our capacity. However, instead of suggesting practicing "doing nothing" in ritualized sessions, I am in favor of developing a relationship with the normal pauses that occur between activities. It can really be that simple. Instead of jumping from the end of one task to the next, become aware of the natural space that forms between the tasks. Look around and notice the different patterns of light flowing around you. Feel your breath and your body without needing to modify anything. Hear the sounds around you or just allow emptiness to emerge. This simple practice is profound, incredibly nourishing, and can be life-changing. If anything, it energizes you because it allows your nervous system to recharge, thus giving you a higher amplitude when you engage with more doing. There is no set number of times to do this or set times frames. Some pauses can be short and others can be substantially longer. Allow the pause to organically emerge and you will find your rhythm.

These pauses can also happen in movement. As you walk from your car to the grocery store, allow yourself to pause by becoming aware of your steps and leisurely make your way to the entrance. Saunter and meander in your path. When you stop at a red light, take that as an opportunity for a pause. When you finish eating, or brushing your teeth, or exercising, simply stop for a moment and take it in. Pausing is a subversive act of rebellion in our culture as we are pressured to always be on. Once this pattern is set, which might be difficult at first, there will be no turning back. In light of contemporary culture, it is a radical shift in how you live that satiates a deep need within.

Pausing helps you tune into a way of life more aligned with that of our deep ancestry from the human to the non-human, and brings us closer to the organic movement of the natural world. It is the culture we now have that swims against the currents of nature. You will find that somehow everything still gets done, and that you have more energy and a clearer mind. If anything, pausing appears to magically create more time. I invite you to harvest the pause and enjoy these natural spaces.

The Inner Worm

The cranial brain is widely accepted today as the seat of consciousness that controls life. While there is a spark of truth in this, it will not light the way to the whole truth. Underneath the capacities of the cranial brain are other centers of intelligence - other functional brains. These seats of consciousness have been validated by contemporary science, and their approaches have also validated their awareness and sense of self also exist. At present, we can point to three orienting places of personhood inside ourselves: the cranial brain, the heart brain, and the gut brain. These brains can actually influence our decisions, remember experiences from the past, and release neurotransmitters. These three centers also happen to be most commonly referenced portals of awareness found around the world in energetic and spiritual traditions. While it is wonderful that in some circles, awareness is descending back into the viscera to encompass more of our totality, it is also an unconscious sleight of hand that the gut and heart are often referred to as the 2nd and 3rd brains in complementary research. From an evolutionary point of view, this is inaccurate and reflective of our obsession with the head. The gut is the first brain, the heart is the second, and the cranial brain is the last in the evolutionary chain.

Some of the first life forms on earth were little more than mobile digestive tracts; worms using their mouth as their primary sense organ and exploring the ocean through mouth-directed movement. Your digestive tract is in many ways a much more complex version of this basic worm, and in reality the same could be said about you as a whole. At your center is one continuous, unbroken tube, from mouth to anus, which undulates and pulsates with its own rhythms; and it is at the core of your physical body. Author and movement expert, Simon Thakur of "Ancestral Movement" likes to refer to it and its impulses (which, in fact, *are* your impulses) as the "inner worm." Your heart and intestines are quite intelligent in a very instinctual and primal way. The heart has a lot of wisdom to share, but for the purposes of this work, we will put more focus on activating the intelligence of the gut.

The intelligence of the gut is especially linked to deep ancestral currents. It is an ancient brain and is perhaps the oldest source of intelligence in the body. Understanding that your guts are a fundamental piece of who you are is a potent step in moving towards a healthier relationship with the deeper ancestral mysteries. Within this gut complex there is also the vagal nerve, which is the largest nerve in your body, and it is a major player in your autonomic nervous system. It innervates all your major organs, and it is especially connected to the gut. The most intriguing fact of this to me is that communication highways are 70-80% upwards! So the gut speaks to the head more than the head speaks to the gut.

Just as your heart has rhythms and can have arrhythmia, so can the gut with its digestion-promoting undulations. It is believed by some researchers that an arrhythmia in the gut is at least partly responsible for diseases like Irritable Bowel Syndrome. Another fascinating tidbit is that over 95% of the serotonin levels in your entire body are located in your intestines, yet modern psychiatry has yet to account for this fact in their perceptions about mental health. The gut brain is a valid source of intelligence, and gut feelings are literal messages coming from a very instinctual and old neural network. Learning to increase the communication between this network and our other brains can enrich many parts of our lives. The next exercise I will share is a potent way of doing this.

There is a lot of trauma and pain stored in the guts for many of us today, and this is a big part of the reason that the heart is brought in to mediate the process. Working with this exercise consistently can open many doors that over the long haul can radically shift awareness. I would go as far as to say that without activating this primal awareness, much of the other work in this book may land as superficial window dressing. It is important to understand that external activities, while valuable, are simply roads into internal, qualitative changes in our perception. It is possible to arrive at these places to some degree with other elements of this book; but this next exercise will provide huge boons for the work of connecting to the ancestral, now. In other words, we can crawl on the ground until our hands bleed and that might get us heading in the right direction. But finding ways to bypass the deep conditioning and wounding that has stripped us of our innate, animal sense of the world is extremely helpful. We go straight to the primal with this practice.

Activating Primal Consciousness

While this exercise can be performed just about anywhere, you will get quick and more effective results if you do this outside, in a relatively wild setting, in no or minimal clothing.

1. Find a place to sit or lie down comfortably and close your eyes or soften your gaze - whichever feels right for you.
2. Now, pay attention to your breathing without attempting to change it.
   If you can, observe the shape of your lungs. Feel the container that is your body. Feel your pelvic floor; your belly; back; ribs and chest. Simply feel.
   Where is your breath moving?
3. Now sense your connection to your environment.
   Feel the pressure of your sit bones on the ground. Feel your hands on the ground or on your thighs. Feel your clothing on your skin (or lack thereof). Listen to the surrounding sounds. Feel the temperature. Feel the place where your inner awareness and the outside world merge.
4. Place your attention in your thoracic cavity and now place your dominant hand on your heart. Feel a gentle magnetism between your hand and chest, and begin to pulse your hand on and off your chest organically, in whatever varied rhythm that naturally emerges. Do this until the intelligence of the heart activates, which will usually express itself as feelings of love, gratitude, or joy. Do your best not to coerce this.
   Once the heart is activated, gently do your best to allow it to remain active during the next phases. We will be diving into

the belly, and the belly tends to store intense emotions and/or trauma. The heart can mediate any intense responses here.

5. Now we are going to awaken the intelligence of the gut and shift our sense of self into the belly. Begin by placing your attention to your mouth. Gently and easily feel the insides of your mouth.
6. Then, notice your swallows. Begin to swallow your awareness.
7. Follow your awareness down through your throat and into your stomach.
8. From there, allow your awareness and sense of self to pour through your small intestines, organically moving side to side inside your abdomen.
   Many people project awareness forward, so try to feel backwards towards the spine, in order to find your center, *deep* in the viscera. Allow this process to happen as slowly as needed. With time, it will likely speed up.
9. Move toward your pelvic floor, and once there, feel into your large intestine. Loop around it and move toward your anus.
10. Now, feel the whole digestive tract and *know* that it is a distinct creature. Know that the digestive tract is in fact a giant worm that began its evolution on the ocean floor billions of years ago. Feel this worm come to life. Let your awareness organically move along the digestive tract, and keep a gentle intention to feel the whole tract at once.
11. Once you have a sense to do this, bring your awareness to the center of the belly intelligence where your center of gravity lives. This is generally found two finger widths below the navel. Continue to maintain gentle attention to the entire inner worm while doing this, and continue to maintain the activated

heart. Keeping a gentle smile on your face while doing this can also help. Keep it smooth. Avoid cramping in the quality of your awareness. The quality of your attention needs to remain open, gentle, and loving, even if you encounter intense sensations.

12. Now, once you feel some activation and warmth in the belly, allow a field of awareness to emanate from your belly outward. This may have a dense, hula-hoop quality around your pelvis and lower belly at first. It can also become oceanic in feeling and give you a sense of being immersed in this field surrounding your body.
13. Now feel the whole of the digestive tract, your deep belly center, your expanding outward field, and your heart, all at once. Just *be* in this and allow for your awareness to move between these different elements; however it feels right for you. Spend as much time here as you'd like.

Once completed, go through steps 1-3 again to reorient in the here and now.

CHAPTER 4

A Context for Primal & Ancestral Movements

As a species, we are incredibly diverse movers. Human beings enjoy one of the most mobile and adaptable bodies in the animal kingdom. We can be martial artists, yogis, weight lifters, swimmers, dancers, or gymnasts; we can chase down caribou in the snow, or we can ride rocket ships into space. Our ability to mold and shape-shift our bodies through the medium of space and time is exquisitely varied. Some would say that "movement is life and life is movement." The only readily perceivable difference between a living body and a dead one is the movement of cells, the pulsating of hearts, and the countless rhythms drumming and moving within the living. This quickening within our anatomy distinguishes life.

Our sense of self and the state of our physical bodies are integrally interconnected. Through engaging our movement faculties, breath, and their interconnected expression, we can drastically alter how we experience ourselves - especially if we hold a reshaping intention in the first place.

The body speaks in many ways not directly related to the voice. Sometimes it speaks in whispers; other times in resounding, echoing broadcasts. It always speaks the truth. The expression and quality of the breath, our proportional relationships, movement patterns, rigidness, and tender softness, speak volumes about how we experience our sense of life. This is true in individual human expression, as well as the wider net of living creatures. Could the impulse for life, or the raw consciousness, of a jellyfish be said to be significantly different from that of a human? Both are alive, both experience life... yet the jellyfish experiences life through its unique body, its unique senses, and its gelatinous movement patterns. We experience it through our bodies, human senses, and our diverse movement capacity.

The body has an almost poetic way of expressing our essence, and language leaves behind bread crumbs we can follow. The following are just a few examples of this.

A person who stresses you can be "a pain in the neck."
We may feel as though we "can't stand on our own two feet."
We "stand up for what we believe in."
We do not want to "live on our knees."
We can "grasp the situation at hand."
"The weight of the world rests on our shoulders."
A statement "can feel heavy."
"She carried the company on her back."

We can expand upon these examples if we watch and listen. These types of idioms speak to a knowing that our sense making in the world, and the sensory experience of the body, are endlessly feeding into each-other. What could it mean for us if we took this melded reality into account, and then acknowledged that we are a rather adaptable species?

Beyond our varied movement skills, our posture can range greatly between upright, extended, rotated, tilted, or slumped. These drastic postural variations from individual to individual are unique to humans among the animal kingdom. Outside of those with illnesses, the majority of animals display a pretty similar "posture" from individual to individual. Many of them also display pretty similar movement qualities. Most cheetahs tend to move like cheetahs. Yet we may find someone with a strong open posture, or someone shaped like a question mark, and the way those two individuals move will be very different. The way I have come to understand this is that our animal movement expression has an element to it that is learned and conditioned; it is circumstantial and malleable.

Identity and sense of self can be shaped, and the qualities of the physical are an excellent starting point for beginning this type of work. To engage the tissues and dissolve tensions, restrictions, and the limited reference points stemming from the sitting upright-modern world can be incredibly rewarding. It is not necessary to become an elite athlete. The real need is to engage your body to whatever degree you are capable of, in ways that feed into cultivation of the deeply alive ancestral lineage that is your birthright as a human being.

If you were born 15,000 years ago in a band of hunter-gatherers, hunting, foraging, tracking, running, climbing, digging, dancing, having sex, and swimming in wild bodies of water - in a lineage of countless generations doing the same - your physical experience would be vastly different than the one you have now. I am quite dismayed with the state of much of our contemporary culture and its lack of relationship to the primal forces that have shaped and molded the human body. Especially when I consider that there are people who can meditate for an hour, perform intense rituals, visualize until the cows come home, and yet, cannot enter into a simple, flat-footed squat. To be clear here, the flat-footed squat is one of *the* most fundamental positions of the human body. People explore ancient traditions as sources of knowledge and wisdom without understanding the context they evolved in. People of the past were, by necessity, much more connected to their bodies and the earth than we are as a general population. Their higher states of consciousness, or magical practices, occurred from a strong platform of embodied, vital awareness. It is us, today, who must reverse engineer many of the foundational elements and restore them if we wish to be more whole. This way, the process of deep, embodied physical cultivation leads into, and becomes, the process of expanded awareness.

Primal Movement Patterns

In the world of fitness, terms get co-opted, wrecked, salvaged, and repurposed on a constant basis; and with the term primal movement, it is no different. I personally define primal movement as: the fundamental movements that form the foundation that all human movement is built upon and are easily seen in the movement of human infants. For example, a baby will enter different stages of development that begin to unfold organically, and within these stages express certain movement patterns. Of course, there will be outliers as not every infant will follow this formula. I do not purport that this is an exact science;

I am noting that there is a tendency. If we follow this primal tapestry, we may agree that there are blueprints that form the foundation of our construction and common movements that emerge from that design. In addition to my personal definition, when referencing the word primal, I am using the meaning: prime or first.

In most developmental cases, primal movements occur without prompting. Just as the newly born foul wobbles as it begins to stand for the first time and proceeds to the stage of being able to run, this is in large, how *we* begin to learn to move - through stages that are built *into* us. Every locomotive animal has its own developmental sequence that the majority of its species adhere to. Crocodiles know how to death roll early on in their lives. It is a movement that is part of the fabric of their creation and interwoven into how the crocodile is anatomically built. As human babies move through the developmental stages, they will begin to explore their body's movement capacities by:

Moving their heads back and forth, side to side, and in rotation;
Rolling from their belly to their back, and vice versa;
Rocking back and forth in various positions, as well as rocking side to side;
Kicking out their legs and pressing out their arms;
Reaching with their arms and legs to test their environment and touch what is around them;
They will perform rudimentary pushup-like movements;
They will wiggle their spine, toes and fingers;
Generally, they will begin crawling on all fours;
They will squat or reach for objects to help them stand;
And then they proceed to walking, running, jumping, and swinging themselves from objects.

This is but a small list of movement patterns that could be considered primal in humans. As adults, we can utilize all of these movements and we can also use them in more athletic expressions. A viable option for exploring these natural movements can be found in Tim Anderson's system. "Original Strength" is built on the foundational movements seen in babies - like rolling, undulating, crawling, rocking - and he guides members through these movements, increases their complexity, and introduces variability and load. "Original Strength" has many resources to help adults become re-acquainted with the movements already discussed, in addition to getting in and out of varied positions from the ground and marching in place, which all have deep, ancestral connections.

In the arena of "primal movement", I would highly recommend this resource, as Tim understands the importance of being able to move freely and with the foundation we were given. Primal movements and impulses yoke the body into a unified whole that can move, express itself, and affect its environment. Our inborn movement patterns weave our bodies together at a muscular and neurological level. In this way, the attachment of our limbs to our core will strengthen and test various natural reflexes that unlock our natural strength.

Many of these patterns are not just human movements. The movement patterns emerge from our deep ancestry and can still be seen in other beings such as worms, fish, reptiles, and other mammals. Humans are but one branch of an extended family tree that includes the rest of life on this planet. Evolution builds upon the structures that work, and therefore, in some ways, we are still like worms, fish and reptiles. We have a shared movement experience. There is often a separation of the other animals of this planet from humans, leaving us with a paradigm where there are "people" and there are "animals." We see ourselves *outside* of nature, looking in, instead of seeing ourselves *intertwined* into the fabric of the natural world. I hope that with some recognition of ourselves in the other, an organic empathy can grow for our earthly relatives and we can know that we are human animals, and that animals are people as well.

Primal movement is an organic and accessible way to begin inhabiting this recognition. We are bound together by this shared heritage of dynamism and orientation through movement; many of us move as many creatures have moved for eons. In my experience, getting down on the ground and working with foundational movement patterns can help reactivate a type of root system that firmly anchors certain aspects of our awareness into the physical world. At some level, it is difficult to crawl on all fours without feeling your animal connection to the earth.

Our ingrained movement patterns, both at neurological and structural levels, will affect our base mode of sensing to some degree. Primal movements tap us into our primal ways of feeling. Ways of moving *are* ways of feeling. These ancient and inherited ways help us to orient ourselves in the world. However, many of us in today's world have a new kinesthetic experience: one that involves sitting in front of screens for long durations, disconnecting us from the primal movements that allow us to properly *feel human.* At a practical level, primal movement can be effective in healing and correcting movement dysfunction while simultaneously building a natural, easily maintained, agility. I, for one, have never been more agile than when I took crawling seriously. I successfully tested my agility by capturing wolves and wolfdogs with large fishnets, jumping eight foot fences during emergencies, and repelling down the side of a cliff to rescue a stranded dog.

Many of the aches and pains that manifest in our bodies can be traced back to a shutting down of the connections made by our original movement patterns. Primal movement creates the necessary connections within our bodies that tie our structure into a unified and capable whole. Historically speaking, these connections were made, maintained, and reinforced through the process of *living* (i.e., walking, running, building things, hunting, having sex, dancing, etc.). If you are suffering from chronic injuries or have been disconnected from your physicality for long periods of time, a steady diet of primal movement for a few years might be positively transformative for you. It is due to the fact that our modern world has divorced us, and perhaps traumatized us, out of these patterns, that they can be so helpful. The beautiful thing is, there are so many ways to build these bodily connections. There are many Chinese and Indonesian martial arts systems, several therapeutic models of movement; countless athletic systems of mobility and strength training, and other fitness-based organizations that seek to reactivate these connections. However, most of these systems often require specialized knowledge and, in general, more skill to do the same thing that a solid session of crawling can do more readily.

As I present it here, primal movement is by no means a set of skills we are required to perform to have the capable, and vibrantly alive body of our ancestors. Though they are a high quality starting point, the *internal connections* are what are required for our bodies to experience the ancestral vibrance and aliveness; and those connections also facilitate eliminating the unnecessary tensions we may carry.

Undulations, Pulsations, and Spasms

Beyond the functional patterns that organically emerge as human beings begin to learn how to move, there are also qualitative movement patterns. Some of these patterns have a functional, locomotive purpose as seen in simple life forms such as worms. Unfortunately, these same intrinsic patterns within humans - like undulations, pulsations and spasms - are restricted in many modern cultures, and in some cases, are even taboo. They represent deeper, and more primitive aspects of aliveness. The rippling sensations and expressions are prevalent in exhibitions of sensuality and sexuality - which might explain some of their taboo.

The word, orgasm, is a conjunction between the words organism and spasm. Orgasms are preceded by increases in tension and have subsequent spasms, pulsations, and undulations - resulting in the release of said tension. Alive and ecstatic sex is often thick with these patterns of movement. We don't have to be in the throes of physical passion to exhibit this basic undulation pattern, as without being conscious of it, this movement is working at the core of our being. Within our gut, muscular waves move food throughout our digestive tract, which is referred to as peristalsis.

Many martial arts and systems of energy work have incorporated these wave-like movements and their wiggling characteristics due to their utility in the transfer of power and/or the release of tension. A form of mind-body therapy called "Bioenergetic Therapy", created by the late therapist, Alexander Lowen, places large emphasis on activating these physical vibrations as they help to break up neurotic patterns - patterns that lead to a lack of vibrancy. Utilizing these movements and vibrations in this practice can bring a high-quality sense of aliveness as they wake up numb and closed-off parts of our being. The movements most often occur in the external elements of the body, and with advanced practice, occur in the visceral tissues and organs.

Another important quality to note about these natural movements is that they are often spontaneous in nature. This allows them to bypass the control mechanisms of the upper, mental centers of our being and the restrictive parameters they can place on us. The movements can literally shake us out of our self-imposed limitations. This may be another reason it is taboo to publicly display them in some cultures. It is a layer of control placed upon us that many other species of animals do not have placed upon them. As necessary, other animals can shake, tremble, and vibrate to their spirits' content without having to worry about another animal giving them the side-eye. Let's consider how acceptable it is to see someone at the gym doing a set of pushups versus seeing someone spontaneously and actively trembling, vibrating, or spasming their body to release tension, or for their health.

Learning to allow these natural movements to occur may allow you to have a greater degree of freedom, and if not overdone, they can be quite health promoting. I truly believe that it is for this reason that very animated, healthy and engaged people are often seen as vibrant - they are *trembling* with the very quality of the primal life force that moves through them! If you would like a pretty straightforward implementation of these sensations, I would recommend looking into the work of Alexander Lowen; Wilhelm Reich; the Kundalini Awakening Process by Tao Semko; and/or the standing practices of China, collectively called Zhang Zhuang. Although I find that some external catalyst that gradually moves us into a deeper capacity is often necessary, I also suggest allowing oneself to explore deeper, orgasmic waves to occur during sex.

The Human Animal Moves Into Complexity

"Humans are certainly surpassed by many other animals in strength and speed, and they fall short of most apes in arboreal locomotor skills and in pedal manipulative capacity. It is doubtful, however, whether any animal exceeds humans in the ability to construct novel body postures and rapid, smoothly produced sequences of novel postures, such as those that are used in dance, gymnastics, some complex tool-making endeavours, mime and gestural sign languages." - Kathleen Gibson

"I would argue that we have a brain for one reason and one reason only - and that's to produce adaptable and complex movement. There is no other reason to have a brain. [...] Things like sensory, memory and cognitive processes are all important, but they are only important to drive movement." - Dan Wolpert

Simple movement transforming into complex movement is a hallmark of the developmental process and is by no means unique to human beings. Dolphins express this by frolicking in the deep blue, as if for the pure joy of it. They hop, spin, flip, and somersault both in and out of the water. The exaltation of channeling multidimensional movements through the body can be deeply enriching and is a birthright. We grow not just by doing *more*, but by *being* better. Raw horse power has its value, but in my view, the human ideal is grace, and the fluid expression of innate power.

It is not just in movement for movement's sake, where complexity stands tall, but in its practical utility. I think of the complex structures that are built by congregations of working ants. They are purposeful acrobats, carrying large objects across diverse environments, moving horizontally, diagonally, vertically, and upside down. They create versatile bridges with one another to facilitate the transport of resources. The webs and structures built by spiders are another amazing example. A large part of how spiders make sense of their world is through their web in such a way that the complex net becomes a part of their nervous system. I'm also reminded of the examples already mentioned in regards to our ancient forebears exhibiting complexity through their hunting and gathering patterns.

We see no *real* comparison when we try to compare traversing the natural world, engaging animals in mortal combat, dancing, weaving and crafting, to a routine of bench presses and curls. Our bodies ask us to engage with the world in diverse and varied ways; to move outside of the linear. Some of us have nervous systems more readily capable of adopting complex movements. Others will thrive under the raw pressure of linear movement. Nonetheless, complexity is part of the natural world and hence part of our reality.

Reality, in and of itself, is infinitely complex, emerging from an incomprehensible number of variables. When we embody deeper complexity, we dance with this recognition. Our perspective can become more fluid and malleable as we physically shift and move across multiple vectors, experiencing the world from different postures and positions. Many of us exist in small, repetitive movement-based boxes. In fact, the square housing and clean-cut segmented walls that are characteristic of our architecture, demands we move in more linear ways, when once our dwellings were round or the endless wilderness itself.

To be clear, there is a difference between complexity and complication. Complexity can, and does, facilitate elegant and simple solutions; whereas complication often creates extra work being done for its own sake. Complexity in movement occurs when you have several, different elements coming together to create a synergistic effect where each component feeds into the other, and the whole becomes more than the sum of its parts. Complication throws together unrelated movements that do not feed into one another in a synergistic fashion or contribute to a unified goal.

An enormous part of complexity in movement is the exhibition of spin and rotation in multiple planes of possible movement; and to find rotation and how it can connect seemingly disparate movements in three dimensions. I find it interesting to note that many researchers are confused by the origin of spin and the energy required to sustain it. Our existence is continuously spinning and spiraling. Subatomic particles, the double helix of DNA, the planets, the solar system, the galaxy - it's all spinning. We even see this force shaping seashells, in the forms of hurricanes, and the little spiral at the top of the human skull seen in the pattern of our hair. Spirals move through the body as well, for our femurs are not popped into our hip sockets, but are in fact, twisted into place by our fascia. The arms and torso also carry spiraling qualities within their makeup. Through rotation and spinning, complex movement is introduced to basic linear patterns.

Complexity is not only evident in movement patterns, or the makeup of physical beings, but is a force in nature that expresses itself across almost any endeavor. It has effects on the developmental path; within the complexity in mathematics that allows for technology; or the nuanced, emotional maturity required in relationships. A human baby fundamentally knows how to manage a few, basic emotions, whereas a therapist must dance with many feelings moving within and without them.

We harness the unique ability to cultivate sophistication in some cases where our built-in mechanisms are replaced with refined skills. For example, the average person facing a threat will experience an adrenaline dump wherein the heart begins to race, muscles tense, tunnel vision locks in, and they rely on their gross motor skills, because primal reflexes have taken over to protect the individual in the absence of refined skills. In contrast, a master martial artist will experience an adrenaline *drip*, as their training has allowed them to learn to relax with an abiding and open awareness while under threat. Although it takes quite a bit of training, sophisticated techniques and qualities can be trained and utilized, while gross motor skills are subverted. Not only is this evident in martial arts, but it can be seen in all extreme and elite sports, from professional skateboarding to Olympic bob-sledding. This is where performance drives humans to get comfortable with high degrees of complexity.

Injecting some complexity into your movement will do wonderful things for your nervous system and for the sense of owning your body in the matrix that is space and time. There are many accessible ways to do so. Some primary principles to follow are:

1. Diverse and varied movements, with an element of rotation or spin.

2. Moving across multiple angles and vectors in a synergistic fashion.
3. Complimentary skills that feed into each other.

Thankfully, others have already created vehicles that we can ride into the sphere of complexity! Here are a few different ways that might get you started if you feel the call:

Practicing a martial art.
Learning to skateboard.
Learning to surf.
Learning to BMX.
Dance and improvisation.
Parkour or free running.
Prasara Yoga.
The TACFIT System.

First and foremost, the main reason to learn any of these would be to enjoy it. I implore you to follow a calling to any of these methods of movement complexity. It is in my opinion that if one explores any of these arts or disciplines, and it engages their heart and touches their bones in a way that nothing else has, *that* it is a worthwhile vehicle to explore and grow within. I ask that you not subjugate yourself to *"I must-"*, *"I need-"*, *"-have to"*, *"-got to"* with any of this. Do it because you love to.

The Animals and Elements Within

It is with a connection to nonhuman animals, and the very elements themselves, that we can encounter how ancestral movement can take on a deeper transpersonal trajectory. It requires us to expand our definition of the ancestral, beyond what is merely obvious; and it requires us to extend "what is human" in a similar fashion. Many cultures, medicine-people, and martial art systems have sought to embody the qualities of animals and the elemental forces that makeup the manifest world. We are unique creatures in that we can have the *intention* to shapeshift, engage with, and express the qualities of *apparently*, "nonhuman" movements.

When we *become* water, fire, earth, metal, wood, space, or air in our movement - are we mimicking qualities as we perceive them, or is there a deeper relationship of connection? When we take on the qualities of the tiger, horse, snake, or rooster - are we imitating them, or are we discovering them within us? It is in this set of questions that deeper mysteries of our place in the universe can begin to come to light.

From an evolutionary point of view, movements that are tiger-like or snake-like need to not be coerced, because they exist somewhere deep inside your genetic makeup. At some point in the past, ancestral forces that you are bound to even now, moved much like these animals. As mentioned earlier, we are *still* worms, fish, and reptiles. With this in mind, to move in "nonhuman ways" would be impossible. I believe that there is a much broader scope of "what is human" than many of the narrow definitions we currently get fed in mainstream mono-culture.

The work of Simon Thakur, of the "Ancestral Movement" system, has been instrumental in my personal exploration and understanding of this. I highly recommend looking into his work. We can move like worms, fish, reptiles, and more, because at some level those beings are literally within us. It is not so much that we seek to move *like* them, but more so that we discover their ancient imprint and *allow* these ancestral forces to move *through* us. I touched on this earlier and believe that we can help unleash our inner animals if we pursue this angle.

For me, the elements are a somewhat different aspect of this theme. I see the elements as The Great Ancestors, as we are quite literally made up of them, and they existed before biological life. Our physical bodies are elemental in the ways that we are earth in the form of minerals, bones and flesh; we are air in the form of oxygen and other gasses; we are fire in the form of electricity and heat; and we are water in the form of blood, interstitial fluid, and lymphatic fluid. In the words of Thomas Myers from "Anatomy Trains": "We are the ocean that got up and walked away." We are also space, for within us there are empty cavities most apparent in our sinus, throat, stomach, intestines and lungs.

When we move like earth, can we *feel* how our structure engages with the earth below us? When we move like water, can we find and *tune into* the literal sack of water that we are? How far can this go?

Several indigenous traditions, meditative systems, and martial arts expand into other forces such as lightning, lakes, wood, and the heavens, among others. Where do humans end and where does the rest of nature begin? I am not sure there is a clear answer to this.

Humans are not *in* the universe, walking around like a gamer wearing a virtual reality helmet. At a deeper level, we *are* the universe. The universe could be said to have a sense of humor, because we humans do. It could be said to be intelligent, because living creatures display intelligence. We are as much a part of the universe as gravity.

Ayurvedic medicine holds that anything that can be experienced - from thoughts, to emotions, to sensations, and physical interactions - has an elemental quality to it. At this stage, it may be clear that there is both a literal and a metaphorical aspect to this; but it is nonetheless a functional framework for understanding ourselves. My relationship to my own totality shifted substantially when I learned to recognize the elemental within. It led to years of exploration with elemental forms of physical training - working with the four primary elements as archetypes in movement.

While you can pursue the teachings of Ayurveda, martial arts, and/or indigenous traditions, there are more straightforward ways to begin inhabiting the elements. None of these are attempts at being objective, so much as exploratory. The sensations and qualities are more important than the activities themselves. When we do this, we can begin to embody a deeper, communal relationship with the natural world as we find it within ourselves, and find ourselves within it.

If you are new to these concepts, the following will provide a starting point. If the activities listed are also new to you, I encourage you to look them up as the internet makes that easy nowadays. If something calls out to you specifically, consider finding a valuable resource to learn from.

Water

Qualities: Smooth, fluid, restorative, flowing, undulating, waving, and soft.

Sensations: Thick, heavy, and flowing.

Can be experienced when you feel like you are moving through warm honey; or that you are underwater because your movements feel thick and under the pressure of the water. However, despite these thick and slow sensations, there is a graceful quality and continuous flow to them.

Movements are often circular and not sharp or linear. Here, movement is supple and fluid; it feels juicy.

Water-like Activities: Yang Tai Chi; Wu Tai Chi; Chen Tai Chi; Vinyasa Yoga; Yin Yoga; Slow Joint Mobility; Chaos from the "5Rhythms" system; and many styles of Qi Gong.

Earth

Qualities: Heavy, dense, stable, unmoving, static, slow, rooted, and strong.

Sensations: Earth movement often feels slow and heavy in a manner more linear than water.

A strong connection to the ground is implied. If we feel the foundation of the movement by how it anchors us to the earth itself, and hold that, we can feel earth. If we are amplifying the effects of gravity, either by adding heavy weights, doing slow grinding movements, or consciously altering how our body relates to gravity, this is earth. Earth may also occur from holding positions for long periods of time.

Feeling grounded and rooted is key.

Activities: Heavy and slow weightlifting, or strength training of any form; Hatha Yoga; Isometrics; Zhang Zhuang or static standing postures; and various forms of ground-based exercises. Exercises that teach us to "resist unwanted movement". Primal movement patterns. Flowing from the "5Rhythms" system.

Air

Qualities: Light, complex, ephemeral, and lofty.

Sensations: Air deals with sensations that are swift, agile, expansive, light, and complex.

When you watch air, you see that it is capable of complex spiraling, spinning, swirling, leaping and circular patterns.

Air gives you a feeling of moving with lightness and buoyancy.

Activities: Baguazhang; acrobatics; movement complexes; light ballistics; trail running; light plyometrics; agility training; dive rolling; skateboard tricks; and Lyrical from the "5Rhythms" system.

Fire

Qualities: Explosive, intense, hot, rapid, and purifying.

Sensations: Fire is the most volatile element and can be extremely destructive if improperly handled. Fire is also the source of life; when properly managed, fire is life giving with the potential to offer renewal and purification.

Fire deals with all that is fast, explosive, quick, and high intensity. It feels hot and is enlivening. Fire causes you to sweat. Intensity is either a catalyst for creative processes or a burnout inducer.

Anything that is metabolic conditioning, or is meant to activate the metabolic furnace, is fire.

Activities: High-intensity interval training; Xing Yi Quan; Boxing; intense gymnastics; wrestling; any competition; crawling for extended periods of time; sprinting; Olympic weightlifting; sledge hammer work/training; and Staccato from "5Rhythms".

The elements provide a useful map for training in the different cycles of intensity. In physical movement, it is not always about measuring intensity through metrics, but about having different types of activities to do that express different qualities. Many people get stuck in one element and become a "one-speed athlete" where the intensity/style of their training is always constant. This can lead to stagnation, overuse, and hormonal disruption. For humans, the natural cycles of movement vary in intensity from nothing (at rest and/or lounging), to all out (hunting, defending, dancing, playing), and everything in between.

If we work with an elemental perspective, movement will take on a much more animist feel and will be a day-by-day exploration. I will speak more on animism later in this book - for now, I leave you with these words from Rumi:

> *"Last night I asked the moon about the Moon, my one question for the visible world, Where is God? The moon says, I am dust stirred up when he passed by. The sun: My face is pale yellow from just now seeing him. Water: I slide on my head and face, like a snake, from a spell he cast. Fire: His lightning – I want to be that restless. Wind: Why so light? I would burn too if I had a choice. Earth, quiet, impregnated: Inside me I have a garden and a bubbling spring."*

CHAPTER 5

The Lower Body as a Source of Intelligence

Modern culture is always looking forward and up, drawn to great heights and escaping the confines of nature. At some level, this is due to our incessant focus on the head as "the only means of knowing." A glaring disconnect that is misaligned from our ancestral heritage is the alienation from the vibrant and rich intelligence of the lower body. The intelligence of the hips, genitals, legs, and feet is woefully atrophied and diminished. Just as roots have been sawed away from civilization, they have been severed from our deep sensorial and neurological levels.

Today we wear shoes that draw our feet into an unfeeling slumber. Thick artificial hides and rubber materials insulate a richly sensitive part of our body that is able to perch. We sit in chairs that deprive our hips and legs of the evolved fundamental resting positions that we would experience by sitting on the ground. We no longer roam the varied terrain on foot. For most of us, the days of dancing on bare earth and sleeping on hard surfaces are gone. In all of these areas, we have removed ourselves from the ground and lifted ourselves into the air. This reduces our total personhood in ways that are difficult to flesh out or give names to. In what manner do the legs contribute to the total processing power of the human being? How does this evolutionary mismatch impact our consciousness?

It is common for people who are barefoot to "walk softly upon the earth." They quietly and fluidly *feel* their way as they walk. Once upon a time, this is how we all lived and related to the ground beneath our feet. By sheer necessity we *listened.* Whereas the booted person tramples though like a bull in a china shop, stomping carelessly with no regard for what is beneath them.

I believe that most of us would do well to awaken a more rich relationship to the ground. It is through relating to the ground that the human being gets the type of feedback she would need to fully inhabit her lower body. Of course, I am in favor of accessible and straightforward ways to begin incorporating this into our modem lives. A great place to begin, one that is simple and easy for most of us, is sitting on the ground.

In situations where we are without access to chairs and have to rely on sitting on the ground, we find ourselves in natural resting positions. Positions such as kneeling, sitting on the instep of our foot, sitting cross-legged, sitting on the knees, and more, come into play when we find ourselves sitting on the ground. There are so many natural resting positions and they are common in every culture around the globe. They are a part of the human structure and our nervous system. Resting on the ground provides our bodies with information and feedback that we do not get elsewhere, and introducing the modern shoe and chairs has cut us away from our connection to that earth-feedback system. Philip Beach, author of "Archetypal Postures", wrote:

> *"The Contractile Field model helps us to understand movement. The opposite of movement is rest; one without the other is nonsensical. At rest we assume natural Archetypal Postures. The archetype is the original pattern or model from which copies are made; the best example or prototype of that class of objects. Archetype used in the context of human movement refers to postures that emerge from, and are embedded within, the interaction of many joints and many muscles. Losing access to our Archetypal Postures is a biomechanical peril. We sit on the floor in many postures that are our birthright, postures that our modern society neglects to value, instead preferring chairs and sofas. Rising from these Archetypal Postures to our full upright bipedal posture uses deeply embedded patterns of movement."*

Inspired by our ancestors, who spent a lot of time on the ground, I suggest we find an excuse to spend time on the ground on a daily basis so we can develop our connection to our lower body intelligence. My recommendation would be to aim for five minutes per day, at first, and then work towards extending that time on the ground to 20 minutes or more. I believe that this can organically occur in everyday activities, rather than attempting to create an exercise session to get on the ground. Applying the mentioned resting positions to your daily life will be so good for you as it immediately adds a low-bandwidth form of grounding to your system.

Here are a couple of ideas to get you started in your exploration of resting on the ground in natural rest positions:

- While watching TV, sit on the ground and play with different leg positions.
- Standing desks are all the rage these days, but I would like to see more desks lower to the ground so one can sit on the ground while working. It might be useful to sit on a cushion at first, but give sitting at your coffee table , perhaps while reading an article on your computer, a go.
- Anytime you are about to sit in a chair can be considered an invitation to explore a ground-based sitting position - even if it's just for a few breaths.
- If you are out and need to take a rest, and if you are capable of doing so, I would encourage you to get on the ground. Kneel on the ground, sit cross-legged, and take a breath.

Another way to tap into our lower body intelligence is by going barefoot. As much as possible, and with gentle transitioning, explore being barefoot outdoors while walking on natural terrain. If this is not feasible, I encourage you to try minimal footwear to explore the outdoors through your feet. Feel your feet in this process. How do they feel? Are they stiff? Are they weak? For those of us who do not make regular practice of moving around barefoot, chances are they will feel stiff or weak. I repeat, gently transition into being a barefoot creature more often. Just simply doing physical training in minimal footwear or barefoot could spark some massive changes in your connection to your lower body.

The Pelvis and Genitals

Our entire lower body has an intelligence field from the pelvis down to our feet. Some might say that everything from the diaphragm *down*, is a matrix of "lower intelligence". Just as the connection to this field has been cut off at the feet, the overwhelming majority of contemporary humans are shut down to the awareness of this field in the hips, pelvis, and genitals. Through my observations of indigenous peoples, I've noticed that they orient themselves through their lower centers more than those in "civilized" society. Due to being more tuned into their lower bodies, they carry themselves "lower in the saddle," if you will. In contrast to the head and heart centers, the lower centers often act as centers of power, grounding, athleticism, free expression, sensuality, and sexual vitality. These aspects of our body, these raw and awesome creative forces within us, literally bring life into existence. Yet, it is these forces that tend to frighten those who are incapable of healthfully integrating the intensity of these centers, and this often leads to the perceived need to shut it down in others through conditioning, physical tensions, and cultural manipulation.

The genitals naturally carry a profound charge within them. In our culture, to be profoundly activated within this region can be quite intimidating. It can often feel dangerous, explosive, or all-consuming. You may have an inkling of what I am referring to in terms of intensity if you have felt the sensation of strong arousal. Many people look for ways to discharge the buildup of energy in unconscious ways. It's often done in unconscious ways because the ability to be *with* these powerful sensations, without feeling ravaged by them, requires deep grounding and a strong internal framework that can support it.

The genitals can act like homing signals - leading us toward the circumstances, people, and activities that invigorate us in life. Desire is the very drive of life itself, encouraging living creatures to rise towards the sun and grow. When we begin to free up intelligence in the pelvis, hips and genitals, we deepen into a greater sense of embodiment of ourselves. I also believe this deep sense of embodiment makes it harder for others to coerce us. Whether conscious of it or not, many of us can recognize those who possess the trait of embodying open and mobile hips. The aliveness that emanates from this area in an individual with such traits is strongly magnetic. Imagine carrying a high degree of energy in your lower centers without being overwhelmed or feeling the impulsive need to discharge the energy, and instead, finding it possible to stay connected to the energy and be guided by its power.

In the broader scope, however, many of us have to take into account trauma and/or wounding within these areas when engaging in this part of ourselves. There are any number of traumas that may be present within this area of our bodies, and if it were needed, a few lines in a book is no substitute for qualified assistance. Outside of the context of serious wounding and sexual trauma, the following exercises are generally safe and gentle for most. There is much more that could be said about the intelligence of our genitals, hips and pelvis, as well as the many layers of releasing, strengthening, and fully engaging these parts of ourselves. The following is a starting point, but the real value will come from consciously inhabiting these areas and allowing their nonverbal form of intelligence to impact our consciousness.

Pelvic Bumping

Lying on your back (on a mat) with knees up and feet flat on the ground, place your heels about 18-24 inches from your glutes.

Gently lift your pelvis up off the ground, about 10-18 inches, and then let it drop onto the ground. This will send a vibration through your pelvic region.

Continue to lift and let go for 5-10 minutes.

In general, what will happen is a natural awakening where the pelvis will try to take over and move however it wants to. You *may* experience waves of pleasure during this exercise. If you can, allow for natural movement and expression to emerge as it wants.

When you are complete, I highly advise that you spend an equal amount of time in stillness and quiet. Feel all of your feelings during this time. This may seem simple, but I can attest that this can be an incredibly powerful practice.

What is turning you on?

In what areas of your life do you get a real sense of aliveness and energy? Consider the different activities, decisions you have recently made, and the trajectory you find yourself on.

Do any of these areas correlate to the aliveness and zest that can be felt in your genitals or pelvis? Be gentle and do your best to feel into this area as you contemplate this question.

This is about learning to work with this area of our body as a homing signal that guides us toward deeper aliveness and pleasure in our daily lives.

Becoming more conscious of the hips and pelvis as you walk.

This is an opportunity to explore the origins of some of our feelings around self-esteem and confidence.

Can your hips and pelvis be more involved as you walk? Can they freely sway side to side, or do they feel stiff and rigid? How does the freedom or stiffness in this area make you feel overall? Is there an effect on your mood and energy? Do you feel confident, afraid, or ashamed as you explore this area of your being?

Ground like a Lightning Rod

"Has the quality of having one's feet on the ground lost its meaning? I believe it has. The modern individual is more properly described as "flying high and fast". It is hard to slow down when the world is racing by. It is difficult to be grounded when the culture itself is ungrounded, when it denies reality and promotes an illusion that success represents a higher state of being and successful people live richer and more fulfilling lives. All the same, the real values of life are "earthy" values: health, gracefulness, connectedness, pleasure and love. But these values have meaning only if one's feet are planted firmly on the ground."

- Alexander Lowen, from "The Spirituality of the Body"

As we descend into the intelligence held within the lower body, we arrive at the bastion of grounding; of being held by the earth. Being grounded is a part of our heritage and it is a baseline element of being human. The majority of our ancestors were grounded beings. When you live in nature, circumstances place you firmly into the reality of the world around and beneath you. Your presence is firm, as to be disengaged from reality for any significant period of time likely leads to injury or death. Today, it seems that being disconnected from the ground is virtually a cultural practice. Distraction, over reliance on the head, a lack of physicality, and a lack of contextual awareness is pervasive. Tension, stress, and trauma further unplug us from our roots.

There are a variety of possible expressions of grounding, especially when we take into account the physical, emotional, mental, and spiritual applications of grounding. At the core level, what does "being grounded" really mean? Fundamentally, grounding is a process of becoming stable, and being grounded means that we are being anchored in such a way that we are *capable* of cultivating stability. As much as we may be detached from our grounded roots, we have an inkling of what grounding means to us. For instance, we inherently know that routines provide a sense of grounding through its consistent rhythm of stability. Even some of our language alludes to this when we say that a person, job, or routine "grounds us;" and we know that when someone or something is "up in the air," that the opposite of groundedness is true.

One of the primary goals of this book is to provide a type of grounding that extends into our experience of life itself; through finding anchors in the stabilizing reality of being a human. The ancestors are *in* the earth and we *are* the earth. The ground is nourishing and calming, and yet, the ground can be energizing. Grounding provides us with the platform from which we can create power; a base from which we can express power; and an anchoring point where we can stabilize power. There is a saying in martial arts that depicts this - "*You* do not hit the person; the *ground* hits them through you."

Grounding also provides us with the ability to manage our levels of charge. For instance, the rise of energy through the body from the ground up, and its movement back down, is a recognized pattern in many energetic circles, because it creates a circuit of energetic exchange. Excessive charge that is unable to move back downward creates overwhelming sensations that need an outlet; and energy that cannot move upward leaves us feeling flat and fatigued. If you are not in touch with the ground, energy moves upward into the shoulders, neck, and head. The breathing begins to come from high in the clavicles, instead of low in the belly, and the person becomes restless, anxious, and comes off as "heady" or "hung up." The ground gives us a touchstone that we can release into when we feel overwhelmed.

For those of us engaged in lofty, spiritual pursuits, grounding allows us to bring our higher realizations into actuality. It is too easy for many spiritual insights to remain heady, ghost-like projections, as opposed to embodied, physical changes in the world. For instance, all of the ancient wisdom traditions of the past emerged from people who were substantially more grounded than we are today just due to *how* they lived. I believe that most of the ancient spiritual practices of the past cannot be taken out of that context. Ancient peoples lived much closer to the earth; they knew the earth to be a living being; and they felt the elements as an immersive experience. It was known to them that life occurred on, and came from the ground beneath them.

We can ground ourselves with objects, people, and energetic structures; and we can even find grounding in the divine if we can create a stable connection to god. Here, though, we will focus on the ground below us. Due to the modern world being pervasively destabilizing, practicing grounding consistently is more important than intellectualizing it. We can benefit greatly from learning how to *sink* our consciousness, as much as raise our consciousness. The following exercises focus on different elements of grounding and can be very effective. You can work with just one of the three exercises or combine them all as one full grounding practice.

Exercise 1

Orienting:

Stand erect with your feet about shoulder-width apart.

Focus on the body, slowly moving from the head down to the toes. Focus on the sensations as you do this. Notice the thickness and heaviness of your mass. Take inventory of what feels light, heavy, disrupted, smooth, hot, cold, etc.

Focus on your breathing. Feel the natural, wave-like flow as it moves in and out of your nostrils, without trying to alter it.

Then, focus on the ground beneath your feet and feel the earth pushing up against you and supporting you.

Begin to lightly bounce while remaining flat-footed, or by coming up on the balls of your feet and then allowing your heels to drop. This will help to reinforce a connection to the feet.

Pause.

Then take a good look around your environment and take it all in. This will let your nervous system orientate itself into your environment. Slowly move your eyes around, naturally allowing your vision to take in the different colors, shadows, light patterns, textures, and qualities of the world around you.

After moving through this exercise once, allow yourself to freely flow between each of the steps again, and repeat as many times as you'd like.

Exercise 2

Feeling the Legs:

Turn your toes in slightly so that you are a little pigeon-toed.

Bend forward at the hips and let your hands hang comfortably *just off the floor* with your knees slightly bent. (**Note:** The legs should not be straight.) Place all of your weight into your legs.

Many people have a tendency to keep their head up in this position. Allow gravity to gently release your head and neck down toward the ground.

Let the weight of your body fall forward onto the balls of your feet. The heels can be slightly raised if needed. Ideally they would stay flat.

Stay conscious of your breath, allowing the breath to go in and out through the nose.

Now, slowly begin to straighten the knees until the hamstring muscles at the back of the legs are stretched. (**Note:** Do not fully lock your knees. Keep a slight bend, or softness, at the knees.)

Try to hold this position for three to five minutes in an intuitive and gentle manner. It will create a very strong set of sensations in the legs.

Exercise 3

Melting:

This is best done from a stance that is narrower than shoulder width.

You'll want your feet, legs, and hips to be aligned so that your skeleton naturally supports your weight.

Feel your weight evenly distributed through all four corners of your feet. Keep the toes pointed forward or very slightly pigeon-toed.

Now, bring your awareness to the top of your head and move it down your body to your feet, while holding the intention of melting all the tension you hold. Imagine the tension releasing from head to toe like hot butter - warm, soft butter; simply releasing down your body and into the ground.

Feel free to make an audible sigh as you do this to help aid the relaxation process of this exercise.

Let your eyes soften. Let them feel heavy, as they do when you get sleepy.

Release.

Some people find it helpful to imagine they are underwater with a pressure that builds as it surrounds them to help them release.

Ideally, by the end of this exercise, it should feel like you just got out of a hot tub, with all of the meat of your body feeling like they are hanging loosely on the bones.

Note: This exercise can be very effective at releasing so much tension that you may find yourself needing to put in a little effort to keep you standing erect.

Reclaiming Wildness through Direct Experience

"What is needed is self actualization not self image actualization."- Bruce Lee

"It is only by grounding our awareness in the living sensation of our bodies that the 'I Am,' our real presence, can awaken."
- G. I. Gurdjieff

The most useful bounty that can emerge from movement practice lies within our internal spaces. Up to this point, there has been a focus on external methodologies and ways of orienting with them; however, the real query is within. The whole of the ancestral movement map is already inside of us and the changes we seek can be facilitated by the practices of movement; but changes that we want are not the practices themselves. To externalize this process is simply another way we commodify our experience and turn something intrinsic into a fetish.

With the aid of ancestral movement, changing the quality of our direct experience is where we can find the most value. By direct experience, I mean a state in which we engage with reality directly, bypassing as much of our filtration system as possible. This is a state where *being* itself is understood as the root of experience; and the body that is *experiencing* is understood as a self-possessed, divine expression of nature. One of the most corrosive, contemporary, inner restrictions that dominate us today, is the eroding of our capacity to experience various layers of reality directly.

The process of re-engaging with the physical through the spirit of the ancestral can lead us deeper into the reclaiming of sovereign, innate-being. This place of direct engagement with self, and the reality we are immersed in, is wildness itself. To be wild is to be self-possessed. The fitness world is replete with false idols, domesticated ideals, arbitrary standards, and superficial methodologies. Why even engage with ancestral or primal movement patterns? Exercising because institutions tell you to, or because peer pressure squeezes your social status, only further separates you from yourself. Every session becomes something that can further sever you from *you*. Improving your health only has value if you want to do something worthwhile with your newfound sense of aliveness: to adventure; to serve; to love deeper; to express more; to increase your depth of being, to align with destiny. Does your new energy simply pour into your restrictions, tightening them around your breath, sensations, or ability to be present with your experience? If this work is not in service of more freedom - of your wildness - then I invite you to consider the point of it all.

Modernity is engineered to impose some degree of existential inhibition that leaves us devoid of the nectar of direct experience - which is to simply *be* a creature on earth who breathes, senses, knows, and moves with grace and dignity. The quality of being present within oneself is something wild animals possess, but that is becoming progressively sanitized. How most of us choose to engage with life is not often influenced by our *actual* experience of living anymore. We have progressively become more conditioned to be less engaged with our own sensemaking in order to be domesticated. Domestication is the process by which an animal has its freedom slowly taken away from it, by having what it can feel, eat, and do, tightly regulated. Its breeding, movement patterns, and energy are subjugated. Its impulses and inner knowing are removed as much as its direct experience is withheld from it. Society is like this, and this has been happening to us since before we were even born.

From the moment we can speak, walk, and act within this civilization, countless forces tell us that what we feel is wrong. We are not taught how to *have* a life; instead we are broken-in like a horse who is having its spirit stolen. In order for this to happen, our feeling and orienting faculties must be severed. This psychosomatic surgery weakens us and makes us easier to manage or lead. What we feel is right in the moment is then stifled, blocked, and even punished. Slowly, a distrust of our own experience sets in, and in confusion we search for direction in the domesticators. We say, "Lead us and protect us." From there, we create stories, adopt disembodied ideals, and do our best to maintain the external boundaries we have been told exist - invisible shackles that feel unmovable.

The modern world becomes virtual - existing separate from the living, breathing essence of reality - and the contemporary mind perceives it through a dense cloud of psychic overlays. So many people today live only in their heads. Heads have immense power, but need grounding stations to fully exert it. It is not an exaggeration to say we all must contend with a type of conditioned psychosis. This psychosis is the reality map handed to us by government institutions, parents, schools, and the overall mind-stream of a society disconnected from the deeper realities of the world - dissociated from the body, nature, divinity and consciousness that dwells therein. Instead of pursuing what feels innately right, many are motivated by puritan thoughts: redemption through suffering; being a martyr; self-deprecation; being elite; being "the best;" being the hero; being the savior; and many other imposed roles that take away from what we actually are - divine wild creatures capable of leading ourselves.

One of the most critical lessons the ancestors offer us is how to be wild once again. However, re-wilding must go beyond the *imitation* of our ancestors. Re-wilding must address the *soul* of the person in order to unlock an inner state that is unburdened by civilized notions of what it means to be human. While working with the wolves, I learned that *being wild* was a quality they possessed regardless of the fact that they were stuck in an enclosure - unable to roam the wilderness to their heart's content. Their external circumstances did not drastically affect that particular innate quality, though. Wolves raised by humans were more willing to be reasoned with, but they certainly could not be commanded or have their sovereignty contained. They did what *they* felt like doing, and relationships with them occurred on *their* terms, not ours. Wildness is a state of *being*, not a set of external circumstances. It is only that external circumstances either facilitate or erode states of being over time. This is why domestication happens over generations and not within a single lifetime.

One of the last true refuges of nature that we as modern people can readily access at any moment, is our body and our consciousness. Our bodies, and our primal core of raw awareness, *is* nature. In them, we can rediscover a sense of being wild - of course, if our orienting faculties can circumvent the fences built around them. To become truly free, we must reclaim our experience through a deep sense of embodiment and a non-manufactured engagement with the forces of life. It is more important now than ever to re-attune the thinking, orienting, and perceptual self with the sensing and experiencing creature. It is so important to get our consciousness to conduct itself *within* the flesh.

One of the most profoundly helpful and available ways to do so is through movement, but the caveat here is that the quality of our intention is paramount. A book could be written on how to internally approach physical training with the intention of cultivating our *innate* wildness - not the *idea* of wildness; but that is beyond the scope of this book. However, I can share some principles that may serve as a compass regardless of how your training takes on its outer shape.

1. The primary fuel for your movement becomes direct engagement with the immediacy of your experience.

To do this, we must begin with intention, for what we intend largely determines the quality of our outcomes. The intention to *get* somewhere with your training is a double-edged sword, though. Holding a strong intent to get stronger, more flexible, more mobile, more powerful, or faster during training can become a potent distraction. These quantitative changes can be extremely useful for planning, creating protocols, and *guiding* your movement. However, having these intents during the process itself can simply stunt your progress due to the focus being on an outcome in the future. The hungrier you are for an external goal, the further removed you are from being *within* the immediacy of your movement.

Refining your direct experience broadens the amount of contact you can make with the present moment. You can do this by keeping two things in mind:

- Do not try to recreate past movement sessions, feelings, or performance metrics.
- Do not manufacture expectations of what needs to happen in any movement session.

Conventional intentions are generally pulling away from the immediacy of your movement, because they pursue previous experiences and urge you to impose expectations on how your training should be. In refining your intentions away from past experiences and opening up to what will happen during your next movement session, you can reset your focus on the raw experience of the now. Come back to this refinement of intention *before* you enter into your movement, or when needed during your movement sessions.

2. Notice your habitual patterns around comfort and resistance to change during movement.

In many cases, creating direct change is a challenging prospect. Our conditioning can at times create constraints that require energy, momentum, and a strong will to shift. Often, there is so much infrastructure in place devoted to keeping certain habitual patterns alive, that to dissolve them and emerge anew feels akin to a type of death. Adding to this, modern life conditions us to be loyal to comfort, and to perceive change as uncomfortable.

In regards to change within movement, and the resistance to it, it is more valuable to consider the inner changes as primary, and the external, technical ones as secondary. External, technical changes may include: new systems, new styles, different recovery protocols, new rep schemes, new tools, and new goals. These are relatively easy to adopt and you will find no shortage of this material. Of course, there are methods which are better than others for different goals, and even different people, but these are not always the main stonewalls we face.

Inner changes refer to qualitative shifts in the complexity of who we are, and emotionally and psychologically allowing ourselves to grow and develop in new ways. These are adaptive changes. When inner change happens within you, it is not the same *you* that adopts a new method. This *you* has been stretched into a broader sense of self, more capable of adapting to or creating change. This means that instead of trying new exercises, we change *how we* engage with each and every moment of movement, and even where our awareness is located during our training. If our loyalty is to comfort, or dullness of mind, we will somehow always sabotage our progress into greater freedom.

- **First, notice your comfort habits.** When you move, how do you maintain your comfort? Is it by mentally numbing yourself, avoiding certain ranges of motion, stopping too soon, or doing too much? Are there changes you fear or volatile emotions you would prefer to avoid? Are you avoiding doing what you know you need to because of unconscious shadows sabotaging your intention? Are you overworking, underworking; have too many focuses; scattered; or is your focus too narrow? You may come to find that movement problems are life problems, and life problems are movement problems.

- **Then, explore training beyond your habituated range of comfort.** Mentally open into more sensations, move into places you do not normally move (in a technically sound manner, always), and go a little further with each exercise - stretching beyond what you think is possible. Conversely, learn to hold back more if your comfort is in pushing too hard. Look for the internal struggles preventing you from adopting the changes you know you need, or increase your capacity to feel the uneasy feelings that can come up during training. Learn to stretch beyond your habituated self image.

3. Settle your awareness upon the immediate embodied sensations of your movement, breath, and structure.

There is a tendency to have a third person perspective in movement - as in watching ourselves performing the exercise. We do this to create distance between ourselves and the raw physicality of the experience, or simply from an inability to really focus our awareness. Find a way to enter into the sensations themselves and shift the location of your subjectivity into your direct engagement.

Don't just observe your sensations - *become* the immediate sensations of your movement. This allows you to embody your direct experience. It's really that simple, but this principle can be a difficult one to put into practice. Be gentle, yet firm, with this one, and give your sense of self time to adapt.

4. Discover yourself within the transitions of recovery.

It is very easy to check-out between sets of exercises, and having ways of consciously inhabiting your attention is a potent way to further your engagement. The space between exercises is the valley after a peak. The space between exercises can be a potent arena to leverage, not just for exercise recovery between sets, but as a place to expand our awareness as well.

Here are some ways to become acquainted with the spaces between sets. Try any and all of them in a single session as you feel is right for you. I do, however, suggest giving all of these a try at one time or another.

- **In between sets, perform the 1st grounding exercise - Orienting - from the "Grounded like a Lightning Rod" section.**
  This settles you into your environment, grounds you, and recenters your focus on the immediacy of the moment.

- **Let go of tunnel vision.**
  Allow your eyes to relax and take in the periphery, but maintain a soft gaze so that you are viewing through your entire field of vision, without focusing upon any one object. If your focus narrows, widen it again. Take in the broader view and expand your awareness.

- **Focus-in on the body.**
  Where do you feel tense, stretched, soft, hard, lax, present, or numb? Allow your awareness to cycle. Are you more, or less, present in different body parts?

- **Focus on the quality of your breathing.**
  Simply pay attention to your breath and feel where it may be stuck, free, shallow, deep, rapid, or slow. Simply be aware of it. How does breathing through the nose vs the mouth make you feel? How does bringing your breath into your belly instead of your chest affect your experience?

- **Shake and vibrate.**
  This is something many animals do in order to release tension, increase blood flow, and shake off stress. Aim to make this a

natural response in your training. It will definitely help to press the reset button between sets!

- **Learn to wiggle in order to tune in more.**
  When tensions rise, or discomfort forms, wiggle it out. If your internal organs feel a little restricted, wiggle your torso. Can you feel your organs? Wiggle your legs. Wiggle your neck.

Apply these principles regardless of what you do and feel the quality of your engagement with life change. Combine this work with ancestral and primal movements, and you will really be cooking with fire.

CHAPTER 6

The Way of Ancestral Nutrition

"The most radical, subversive thing you can do, the thing that will pour sand in the gears of the Vast Machine, is to take back control over your food. Buy your food as basic ingredients, cook them yourself and eat your meals with family and friends"
- Mushtaq Al Ali Ansari

"Food for us comes from our relatives, whether they have wings or fins or roots. That is how we consider food. Food has a culture. It has a history. It has a story. It has relationships."
- Winona LaDuke

Through the winding tributaries and shifting currents of the ancestral, we now transition into one of the most difficult topics to contextualize in a manner that is living, dynamic, and relevant to modern people: ancestral nutrition. This section outlines what I have come to experience as the *practice* of being a hunter-gatherer in the 21st century. A simple truth must be established as a platform for everything that follows from herein: **nutrition is deeply personal**. Regardless of how cultivated our skills, or how advanced of a practitioner we are in other domains, it is likely that our response to certain foods, meal timings, sources, or preparation methods will force us to simply stop, listen, and *follow* the mystery of our body's intelligence. Yes, science has mapped out various fundamental layers of digestion; but when we consume something, a deep and ancient wisdom takes over and our body acts like a discerning, nuclear reactor - simultaneously coordinating numerous internal combustions, while spontaneously weighing a multitude of needs. We may know the mechanics of digestion, but there is an enigma about the process. It is a wonderful, beautiful, and for some of us - at certain times, terrible event. Nutrition is one of the most innocent expressions of the wild, and at times, uncontrollable nature of our body.

At first glance, it may appear that this section relates specifically to how we eat, or even *what* to eat. If you were hoping to be converted here, you may be disappointed as I have no desire to point you to any particular dietary pilgrimage. Nutrition is an arena where many "leading authorities" want you to worship their particular dietary religion. I believe that we must take personal responsibility in our relationship to food, to self, and to the environment. We must turn down the volume coming from the diverse and ubiquitous "food authorities" in our lives and make sovereign decisions about what we ascribe to here. Suffice to say, I will not present a particular diet for you to follow. Instead, in the spirit of our ancestors, I only want to offer a *way*. Using the principles forged by the human relationship to deep time and bringing them into our modern landscape, I invite us to explore different aspects of the human condition through the lens of food. I hope to broaden our relationship with food beyond what we chew and swallow, and begin to reflect on the deeper belief structures tied to our relation to food, and how it helps us to orient ourselves in the world.

Nutrition has been a very deep passion of mine for many years, and it has led me toward numerous dietary disciplines, ranging from eating one massive carnivorous meal a day, to many small plant-based meals throughout the day, and everything in between. After all of the years of experimentation, as well as in helping a variety of individuals discover their own particular nutritional needs, it is my conclusion that no perfect dietary configuration exists - even for a single individual in their lifetime. How we eat is a living dance. That dance can flow with ease at times, and at other times, it can feel like a bit of a whirlwind. It is meant to change and grow as we do. We do not need diets - we need principles. We need *a way.*

As we move into this territory, I would like to invite you to set aside your preconceptions about the role food plays in your life, because the view we are going to take begins at about 10,000 feet. After the work of narrowing it down, it will be firmly placed in *your* hands. As lofty as it may seem, my primary goal with this section is to provide you with at least one opportunity for a radical shift in how you view nutrition. If that occurs, it can change the way you move through the world.

We Are What We Eat

As a species, our relationship to food is fundamental in how we understand ourselves. Even our anthropological designation falls under our food-acquiring behavior: we are hunter-gatherers. Our design holds the charge of hunting and gathering in order to live, and in this way of sustaining ourselves, it orients us in the world; and it gives, and takes away, our options around how much time we can spend on other activities. Eating can be akin to taking a breath, where we inhale the physical world and we exhale excrement. Essentially, without food, we wither and die; and the opportunity to flourish is much closer at hand when we have access to high quality food.

In many ways, our environments have given us what we need to thrive, as many places we have inhabited where plant life is scarce have had many animals to hunt and eat, and therefore nourish ourselves with. Of course, in most cases, we humans are not *strictly* carnivorous. The ability to gather provides us with a wider range of possibilities, allowing us to supplement the consumption of animals. This, in turn, gives us a more adaptable geographical range than pure carnivores, who constantly need large game or an abundance of water-dwelling creatures to survive.

In some cases, gathering has been a dominant and helpful trait. It has made us even more capable of adjusting and adapting to our environmental circumstances. Many have mistakenly compared our human gathering behavior with the behavior and way of being a herbivore, but it is simply inaccurate. No other creature can eat vegetables, fruits, grains, legumes, tubers, nuts, and seeds with the sheer variety, diversity, or quantity that we can. We are not herbivores; we are *gatherers,* and there *is* a difference. Herbivores must spend much of their waking hours eating in order to fill their caloric needs.For example, cows spend six hours a day eating and another eight to chew their cud. Gorillas need to consume 40-70 pounds of food a day and often spend half of their day eating. In contrast, predators exert energy every so often to take down large prey, and lounge and hang around for the majority of their day. A lion can eat one large, 75 pound meal a week and rest for over 20 hours a day. Because of our hunter-gatherer diet, humans have continuously had time and energy available to them to put into other things, such as skills and art.

Our hunting-gathering heritage shaped our dietary flexibility, giving us the time and energy to explore relationships, scout novel areas, perform magic, to focus on our spirituality, and to be creative. In turn, our ancestors began to live a nomadic existence, as they were empowered to traverse and inhabit different regions across the globe. Locations with an abundance of food and water became cultural nodes, attracting human settlements around them like magnets and unifying our ancestors. This unification fostered the ability to cultivate cultural-based ways of eating that offered a sense of collective identity. This still happens at tribal levels, all the way to the scale of modern countries.

A large part of how humans connect to their cultural or ethnic group is through food-based patterns. The areas in which a family lives, and the places their ancestors originated from, influences likes, dislikes, and even the compatibility of certain foods within the body. Many cultures still have a traditional, dietary wisdom to fall back on that does not exist in certain industrialized nations. Different countries have their own unique styles and expressions with food that can change the configuration of the same ingredients used and eaten within other countries. By favoring different spices, utilizing different preparation methods, and having their own flare with presentation, those same ingredients will pop, or blend, uniquely to the country in which it is dished up.

Beyond evolution and culture, the way we choose to eat nowadays can be a reflection of philosophical, religious, and/or devotional aspirations. Consider the yogi who is a vegetarian because of their devotion to harmlessness, or those who subscribe to biblical ways of life choosing to eat based on the dietary model of the Bible. We see this with Muslims who only eat halal food, and Jews who maintain kosher-only dietary habits. In some cultures, food is shared with their gods during special occasions, such as in the celebratory festivals in Hinduism. Within various African Diaspora traditions, the initiated are made aware of certain foods that are taboo for them to eat as it may interfere with good fortune, and those foods that are taboo to share with the gods as offerings. Today, we see the emergence of new, distinct dietary preferences within relatively young cultures, such as those who wander into new age spiritualism, which seemingly gather around "superfood" smoothies and juices, green drinks, and cacao.

The meaning we ascribe to food is an exploration of culture. What we choose to consume, how it is acquired, and the rituals surrounding the act of eating; from the rigid habits of Victorian society to the free-for-all feast of Dionysian festivals, the intricacies of food are forms of communication. Beyond sustaining the capacity for life, food strengthens the bond between individuals, communities, and even countries. In many ways, food can determine family roles, rules, and reinforce long-held traditions. It can also shed light on some of the most fundamental beliefs we have about ourselves and others.

In the proper context this can be nourishing information, but it can also be hijacked, redirected, and used against us. We can see evidence of the power that food possesses as corporations gain control over food culture, leading to a wealth of unhealthy behavior. Let us consider the countless commercials, and carefully crafted propaganda, telling you why you deserve a tasty snack, followed by even more broadcasts about why you need to lose weight in order to be loved. In contemporary dietary circles, the power of food is warped by taking a particular way of eating and transforming it into a religious doctrine to follow, which many end up doing in a desperate attempt to find meaning in a world without any. This is why people seem to love diet books as well as the labels that come with them, or become subservient to the newest study telling them what they *should* be eating. We *want* to be told what to eat, because we *want* to be told who to be. This neurotic need to have our own nature explained to us by outside authorities and institutions who seek to stick all of us in neat little boxes, is a chilling element of the unspoken, yet very present culture of the modern industrialized human. In order to begin untangling some of this, we need to begin broadening our identity and putting our place, here and now, into context.

Creatures of The Earth

First, foremost, and beyond any external culture, each of us are citizens of the earth and its rich history of life. We humans find ourselves at an interesting intersection of time, because we are both creatures *of* the earth and we are also children of the modern space-age. We, as a whole, were born into a world that is very different from the world *we* are in now. Our birthing ground, the earth, gave us inherent needs that are not often met within civilization as it currently stands. As creatures of the earth, our human animal nutritional needs have been shaped by billions of years of evolution, and our bodies *are* billions of years old. This simple truth extends into The Way of Ancestral Nutrition.

Ancestral nutrition beckons us to return to the primal reality that is present within the fabric of the earth. All food, even processed junk food, starts off as a substance that comes from the earth. Processed food goes through stages of refinement, purification, and transformation to become what it is; often to our detriment. It goes through a process of losing its direct connection with the earth - a process similar to what modern human beings have experienced. If we can realize this, and own this as a truth, it may help us ground ourselves into some sense of stability. We can then immediately discard dietary ideas whose genesis depends on a stark disconnect from our past and/or the earth. From that grounded place of knowing, and discarding that which seeks to keep us disconnected, we can then focus our lens on eating whole foods.

In fact, if there was one principle that was central to ancestral nutrition, it would be this: Eat whole foods created by nature. When it comes to consuming whole foods, we are consuming sustenance that bubbled up from the earth's primordial sphere. Certainly, we may have encouraged the hybridization of certain whole foods by planting the seeds and watering them; but *we* did not create the potential found within those seeds. We did not create the life-giving properties of the water or the soil that held the seeds. We did not create the power of the sun that nurtured it into maturity - asking it to rise from the ground. The fundamental properties found within the seed, the earth, and the water would exist whether or not humans intervened. The same can not be said about Twinkies. Although this may seem obvious, sadly, to many it is not.

At one time, gathering food was a rich, grimy, and wild process. whereas these days it is a clean, efficient, and domesticated affair. Blood is no longer spilled onto our hands during a kill, and for many of us, dirt does not need to be washed off our plants before we eat them. We now have rectangular boxes and attractive packaging containing our food. Instead of hearing hoofbeats hitting the earth, or being pulled to brightly colored wild fruits, we see commercials put together by world-class marketing teams trying to get you to buy their product.

In my eyes, the major food companies see us as dollars in their bank accounts. They put unfathomable amounts of money into marketing research conducted by teams of scientists that show them how to craft their products in ways that make them addictive to the consumer. To much dismay, I am often impressed with the effectiveness of their business strategy. Ever hear "Chips: you can't have just one."? That type of response to modern food is not an accident; it's a carefully crafted outcome. *This* is where food ties into a fundamental layer of control and conditioning placed upon modern society. A place where you are *not* free, unless you consciously choose to be.

Humans are drawn to crunchy foods, foods that are sweet; we crave salty foods, and, for the most part, have a desire for meaty flavors - all of which can be, and are, found in the wild. These different tastes signify to our bodies that these foods are nutrient dense and have an abundance of calories to strengthen and/or energize us. Like other animals, and without access to convenient refrigerators, overeating (or storing calories) was beneficial when food was plentiful. However, in today's society, where food is usually easily available and accessible year-round, overeating is a major hindrance to good health. Moreso, easy access to processed and packaged foods are often energy dense, but are lacking in nutrients; whereas whole foods can often layer energy and necessary nutrients by default.

Energy and nutrients are dependent on each other, and a removal of one at the expense of the other can create major problems. Our bodies need the nutrients from food in order to process and use the energy found within it. In the absence of either, such as in diets rich in energy and nutrient poor, the body is unable to use the energy efficiently and that can lead to illness. If we return to simple, whole foods, we can begin to take back control, and ground our relationship to food. It can be a great way to start, yet for many of us, the process does not end there.

Children of the Space Age

As much as we are creatures of the earth, and at one point in our evolutionary history, we crawled out of the same elemental cauldron as the rest of the animal kingdom - we can not ignore where we are now and how it affects our current needs. For most of us are no longer subjected to the different moods of the earth; most of us no longer hunt and gather for our food; and nowadays, we come from a very diverse generational pool. Our ancestors once looked up at the sky in wonderment, awe, and reverence, labeling the sky as the resting place of the gods. How many of us look up now and reflect on the knowledge that we have launched rockets and satellites into the sky and have essentially accosted space?

Our current nervous systems and imaginations have been bred in a climate of technology, electronics, sci-fi storylines, and non-native electromagnetic fields. Our hormones are subject to the wrath of endocrine disruptors that run rampant in our food supply, medications, cosmetics, and water. The elements we are often exposed to are artificial - plastic has replaced clay. Our stress is constant and not acute; our movement is excessively linear and not sufficiently complex; our resting positions are chair-based and not innate. Though our bodies are built on our hunter-gatherer blueprint, there is a big shift in the type of material we are getting for this construction. Our lifestyles, cultural values, world views, spiritual practices, and, dare I say, our very spirits have been systemically stripped of as much of their innate humanity as possible. Although our species-level needs emerged from a broad shared history, as a people, there is much misaligned with that past. Furthermore, generations currently alive can never *fully* go back. Even if we were to drop all the externalizations that keep us tied to society, and move into the bush and live with no assistance whatsoever from the modern world, its imprint would still be with us. We are forever changed by modern times.

So, here we are in the 21st century, as Homo sapiens, caught at a turning point in the known history of humanity. Some of us understand the healing power held in the lines of communication connecting us to our ancestral past. Though some may understand that, *many* of us do not speak the language. While our world spins at light speed, hurtling towards virtual reality, artificial intelligence, singularity, and god knows what, the best we can do is try to create our own dialect. Without connection to the ancestral, we will be like loose buoys in an ocean beyond our comprehension - untethered and afloat to whatever insidiousness lurks under the surface. Without a stable root system, we can be easily swayed by the weak currents of popular media, politics, religious institutions, big tech, public opinion, and the vicissitudes of the modern mind. Put simply, without this stable connection to our ancestors, we are lost. If you do not know where you have been, it is difficult to know where you are going. Food may seem like the least of it, but it is actually one of the places where we can maintain sovereignty with self and ancestors, even if we shop in grocery stores.

A Hunter-gatherer on a Rocketship

Contrary to popular belief, I believe that nearly any diet based on whole foods is "ancestral" with varying degrees of quality being a distinguishing factor. This may be as true for the carnivore as it is for the vegan; even though these extremes are rare from a purely ancestral perspective devoid of the context of the modern world. Regardless of the external form our nutrition takes, whatever we consume is possible because of "The" ancestors and our individual ancestors. With this in mind, I propose a different set of questions as opposed to the question of whether or not we follow some arbitrary selection of available foods that are labeled as "paleolithic", "primal", or "ancestral". Instead, let us ask "What is the overall quality of the whole diet?" and "What is its overall compatibility with the natural phenomena that is *my* body?"

If we no longer actually hunt and gather in the wild as a primary vocation, but seek to consume a diet inspired by this inheritance, then what are we? I enjoy the metaphor of being a hunter-gatherer on a rocket ship to describe the current situation for our ancient bodies in contemporary times. How does our nature change if we consider that we eat like hunter-gatherers, have a territory that spans across the earth;

all the while, spending our days writing, creating sonnets, solving quantum equations, or running a company? To me, having wild game I bought at a grocery store, with fire-roasted, store-bought potatoes for dinner, followed by a video call with a friend who lives on the other side of the world, is an interesting proposition and is a fine example of this.

Nutrition can be such a challenging area for so many of us, especially for those of us currently dealing with health challenges. At some level, we are creating a life that falls outside of any known ancestral context, and yet, it all depends on where we came from. Again, for many of us, there is no clear cultural background to look to. Therefore, I propose we create our own context to help us move forward with our nutritional needs.

Understanding what purpose our dietary strategy serves is increasingly important, as merely surviving is but one layer of relating to food. So with that, I suggest that we ask, "What am I eating for?" For me, nutrition is meant to support what I choose to do and to meet my needs. These needs are at some level ingrained, and at another, environmentally determined. The needs of a modern human are in many ways the same, as well as vastly different from the needs of our ancient ancestors. The needs you have are unique to *you*. No other living thing has the exact set of nutritional needs you have at *this* moment. Your needs are affected by:

your unique ancestry;
where you live;
what season you're in;
what your activity level is;

your work and the *type* of work you do;
what types of activities you engage in;
your health status;
your goals and desires;
your gender;
the practices you have like meditation, magic, or other rituals;
how often you have sex;
how much stress you are under;
the impact of solar or lunar cycles;
and the way your unique body processes certain nutrients.

Your needs will change as time moves, as you are an ever-changing being. If there were a critical truth to grasp here, it would be that how we eat is relational, and that our nutritional needs are dynamically shifting in real time in response to a multitude of variables. Our nutritional needs are not static Reference Daily Intakes given to us by governments or gurus. How we get those needs met can *only* be done one meal at a time.

CHAPTER 7

The Impulse to Thrive

If there is an overarching intention ingrained in all living beings, it is to thrive and to flourish. This is an ancestral inheritance that extends far beyond humans and moves as far back as the origins of life. You can witness it in the tree that blossoms forth with fruit, or the bull that expresses his full size, grace, and power. While nutrition can have many uses that include social, religious, or cultural purposes, and at times, can be worked with as a form of medication, the most profound purpose it can uphold is to support thriving. Thriving can encompass any and all of the previously stated uses of food at different times. This is nutrition expressed in the ideal; and we must, of course, acknowledge that "the ideal" is not always possible. Yet if it is possible, I assert that it is our responsibility to dance with that possibility.

Every species seeks to blossom to the best of its ability given its available resources. While thriving requires an abundance of resources outside the scope of food - nutrition, in this case, is a major resource. Just as the tree needs rich soil, sunlight, air, space, and the appropriate climate to burst forth and bear its fruit, a hunter-gatherer on a rocket ship requires nutrients and energy to thrive. The hunter-gatherer also needs social connection, the ability to move and to express itself, to love, to learn, and to grow. How can food support this? Let us expand on the idea that food relates to thriving with a look at multiple layers of eating through the following model. I hope it is useful for you.

The Four Layers of Eating

Layer One - Basic Survival:
This layer of eating is based purely on the impulsive patterns that supply enough caloric intake needed to stay alive. Unfortunately, there are many cultures that are forced into this form of eating due to a lack of resources and the erosion of their traditional ways of life. In many nations, whether they are developed or underdeveloped, many people have to eat with basic survival as their default layer due to poverty and other factors. With whatever is available to them, they will and can survive on anything that provides their caloric needs, and the quality of food can range from junk food (highly processed, often cheaper) to high-quality foods that can be accessed. Plain and simple, layer one means that our main reason for eating is to stay alive. It is possible that any of us could be pushed into this level of eating at some point in our lives. When our main concern is simply not to starve, then our decisions change about what is acceptable to eat.

Layer Two - Over or Undereating:
When there is a surplus of available food and basic survival is not threatened, overeating can occur more easily. With this layer, there can be a tendency toward unconscious patterns of eating as the attentiveness to the actual *need* of the body is not the primary focus. Some unconscious patterns can include numbing oneself with food, substituting food for other hunger drives in life (like addictions), eating

excessively due to dysfunctional behaviors learned from childhood, etc. Within this layer, the fear of not having enough can lead to overeating. Just as surely as our bodies can not thrive without enough food, our bodies can be destroyed by having too much food - it is often just a much slower path to death.

On the opposite side of the spectrum of this layer, we have the less common layer of undereating. There may be a disorder in which pathological factors may be at play, but undereating can also occur in more subtle ways where there is little priority given to nourishing oneself. There may be an over-reliance on stimulants or other drugs that blunt hunger. In this case, food can be easily accessible, but the drive to nourish oneself is either consciously or unconsciously shunned.

Layer Three - Functional:
This relates to an explicit purpose separate from longevity, survival, dysfunction, or impulse. Here, one is eating to accomplish something specific. The most common example of this is to eat for athletic performance, muscle building or cutting to fit into a specific weight class, or for appearance-based purposes. Another example of functional eating would be eating for the energy to accomplish specific tasks or to get through a particular event. Relating to food as medicine to potentially ease or cure a particular disease can be seen as functional. This layer of eating is working with food to accomplish something specific in a clearly defined and directed way.

Layer Four - Thriving:
Eating with the intention of thriving includes superior health, longevity, and the ability to carry out the myriad of tasks necessary in

one's life, both in the remedial and generative areas. Eating to thrive is a process of self-knowledge and a periodic adjustment to one's daily needs. This layer requires knowing enough about nutrition to make high-quality choices to support us. Here, we want a diet that supports and nourishes our endeavors, and provides an abundance of the necessary nutrients required for this, without supplying more than necessary. It is eating in a way that is ideal for us, and by default, it requires a certain level of ease. However, make no mistake, this level of eating is an ongoing dance and is by far, the most challenging layer to integrate. This is nutrition as a practice. It not only requires self-knowledge; it requires devotion.

In some ways, many tribal cultures who had access to an abundance of food in the varied areas they lived, were eating at this level. Imagine it. Your tribe has hunted and brought home a fresh kill. The whole animal is put to use. Others have brought the wild and local plant life they have gathered for the whole. To me, this seems like an incredibly nutritious and diverse diet that happens to be organic, in season, and even local! Eating to thrive is meant to support fertility and strength - values that are held by many indigenous cultures. Eating to thrive allows us to blossom and express our full potential. To thrive is to live a full life.

If we can agree with, and invite this model of eating into our way of orienting toward our personal nutritional needs, then ancestral nutrition is a call for us to get clear about what the conditions of thriving mean to us. In a time where we no longer exist in tribes that set clear parameters for what flourishing really means, chances are most of us need to choose what that means for ourselves. Once we know what we want is to thrive, the question that can help point the way is: How can food support me to thrive?

Nowadays, provided we have the right resources, we can choose to live in nearly any environment on earth. We can live in Hawai'i, train like a Shaolin monk, medidate like a yogi, perform magick like a Roman occultist, have sex like a rockstar, take psychedelics, and make money helping people grow their business. So many things are possible today. With all of that possibility, we each have to choose for ourselves what the trajectory of our life is going to be. To top that off, we each have our own set of particular health challenges, melting pot of genetics, personal tastes, and budgets. In some ways, hunter-gatherers today are limited to their environment, the seasons that fall within that environment, and their lifestyle. Whereas, some of us can eat special berries that come from Asia, smoked meats delivered from Texas, greens shipped from Mexico, cheese made in New Zealand, and butter churned in Switzerland - and have them all in one meal! All of this to say, it becomes clear to me that there is no perfect diet for all that exists. There is no standard, and relative to scale, this has always been the case.

Avoid Paleolithic Reenactment

I have made a clear intention to resist the nostalgic allure of freezing our ancestors in time, and attempting to reenact their lifeways. If we do so, we lose touch with the living, breathing reality of The Ancestral Now. What we can do is learn, relate, absorb, and discover the ancestral within ourselves. It is due to this that I am often dismayed with the parody we call "The Paleolithic diet" and trying to recreate or re-enact it today. In my opinion, the idea that we even could replicate it, is deeply flawed. For instance, the mantra that echoes within this circle is to "eat like a caveman". It is an inaccurate saying as our Paleolithic ancestors were not primarily cave dwellers. This approach can be beneficial in the sense that it calls out to the past, but we may find that there is no real response reverberating back to us. "The Paleolithic diet" is a neat, little, contemporary package. We cannot, and should not, try to eat like Homo sapiens that lived in the Paleolithic era.

Why? Well, for one reason, many of those foods do not exist today. We cannot imagine the sheer variety of animals and plants that were eaten during that era, which spanned nearly two million years. We know that the domesticated animals and hybridized plant people we eat today were not on the menu back then. We are not hunting down and eating entire mammoths, mastodons, giant cave lions, or giant bears. Paleolithic people were chasing down mega-fauna, and eating plants that grew around them, bathed in the local waters and natural cycles of sunlight of their time. The soil was richer, and more vital. The environment has changed significantly since then. There are pollutants and other man-made chemicals spanning the entire globe that were not around in that era, and which are now a part of our food supply.

Obviously, the Paleolithic ancestors were not eating pre-packaged products like gluten-free coconut macaroons, teriyaki-flavored beef jerky, or collagen-protein powder-cacao-pumpkin seed-bars. They weren't subjected to marketing gimmicks that fit certain nostalgic sentiments and sought to mummify the wondrous relationship between humans and food. Paleolithic humans were not trying to be Paleolithic. They were attempting to survive and thrive, if possible, in a certain time and place. They ate what was available and accessible to them.

Today it seems that in the desire to be like our ancestors, we have forgotten how they might have thought about their situation and have relegated them to a set of temporary circumstances. This faulty meaning-making way of relating to our dietary past creates many forms of dissonance. In some cases, the Paleolithic diet unnecessarily restricts easily available, nutritious, contemporary foods such as dairy, tubers, and legumes, based on the idea that no humans during that era ate them. Even if that were true, which we cannot say for sure, it does not interfere with the possibility that between now and then some humans have emerged that can take advantage of those resources as a food source.

There have been many healthy societies that have been studied to have eaten all of those foods with no apparent ill effects. The questions that we can begin to ask ourselves in relation to these foods are: Do I tolerate and digest legumes well as an individual? Are they a legitimate food source for me in this era? Did my ancestors develop a capacity to digest dairy? Can I consume properly prepared grains with no ill effect?

In general, "the Paleolithic diet" recommends lean protein, vegetables, fruits, herbs and spices, nuts and seeds; all else is shunned. While this may be a high-quality diet, it is by no means authentic - which is the point I am getting at. Regardless of what we eat, or how we prepare it, it is not possible to eat like our Paleolithic ancestors. The Paleolithic era is over and the world is in a different era. The spirits of time have turned the wheel, and if you try to hold on, you will be metaphorically ripped apart.

Learning From Pre-industrial Humans

One of the most worthwhile books on nutrition was originally published in 1939 and was written by a dentist named, Weston A. Price. He traveled the world in the 1920s and 1930s and studied tribal cultures who were not overtly influenced by civilization. He observed their diets, constitutions, and dental health. He found and documented a striking contrast between those who lived on their traditional diets vs. those who started including even a *little* of the modern luxuries of eating. He found that dental health and general constitutional robustness suffered greatly for those who began including refined foods. His book, "Nutrition and Physical Degeneration" includes many photos illustrating the contrasts and his explorations.

When I worked at the wolf sanctuary, we would see this phenomenon often in animals that had been given kibble for many years - much of which were filled with corn, wheat, and other fillers that aren't natural to a canine's diet. They would arrive bloated, suffering from arthritis, and have tooth decay that was more advanced than was appropriate for their age. As they transitioned to an all meat diet, even one that was imperfect by wild standards, many of their symptoms would improve. In many ways, humans on modern, refined diets are much like these wolves and wolfdogs we cared for.

The study of pre-industrial people and modern tribal cultures has more to offer about the impact of nutrition on health than does the theoretical frameworks of a plausible Paleolithic dietary past. It is even possible to sit with, and share a meal with, these living people instead of the fossils of the Paleolithic era. Dr. Price found pre-industrial, tribal people to be healthy, robust, lean, fertile, and strong. Of course, this was due to much more than diet alone, but nutrition did seem to play an important role. Many of these healthy, living cultures ate things like grains, legumes, and dairy. They also ate simple meals with a high organ-to-muscle meat ratio, roots, tubers, wild fruits, vegetables, insects, honey, seafood, and various terrestrial and water plants. There was a big emphasis on eating the whole animal through the use of bones, cartilage, and gristle. Of course, it is likely that Paleolithic people also ate this way, but with what they had available to them.

There is no Single, Ancestral Diet

Akin to the mishap of trying to isolate a Paleolithic diet, a lot of different dietary circles make claims about what the ancestral diet was and present blanket statements that do not hold up to the fires of scrutiny. A distinguishing characteristic of ancestral diets is adaptability. This is obvious from the diversity of places humans have inhabited on this planet. Is the ancestral diet of people living in the Polynesian islands the same as those living in northern Europe?

To further our exploration of pre-industrial dietary territory, and our closest approximation of ancestral diets, here are some examples of what Dr. Weston A. Price discovered tribal people eating:

The Swiss of the Lötschental Valley:

- Fresh, hand-milled, rye bread.
- Raw cheese, butter, and milk from cows eating fast-growing alpine grass, which supercharged the dairy with vitamins.
- Fresh and preserved, local vegetables.

The Native Americans of the Rocky Mountains:

- Organs and bones of game animals, with a heavy focus on moose and caribou. Muscle meat was often fed to the dogs and considered sub optimal for human consumption. *(So much for those tasty steaks or Buffalo burgers!)*
- Bark, tree buds, and other vegetation, much of which was only available in the summer.

The Gaelic in the Outer and Inner Hebrides:

- Seafood including oysters, fish, lobsters,crabs and clams. Cod liver was particularly valued.
- Fresh vegetables in the summer; stored vegetables in the winter.
- Lots of oats in the form of porridge and oatcakes. They practically had oats at every meal.

Tribes in Eastern and Central Africa:

- An abundance of sweet potatoes, beans, corn, and millet.
- Water plants, fish, and shellfish.
- Game animals.
- Domesticated goats and cattle were raised for their meat and dairy.
- Insects, like ants and locusts, were eaten in a variety of ways.

The Eskimos of Alaska:

- Animals of the sea in their entirety - the fat/oils, their skin, and organs.
- Caribou and other land animals.
- Fish and their eggs.
- Vegetation gathered in the summer months and preserved for the long winters in seal oil.

South Sea Islanders:

- Nutrient-dense diet of seafood of all sorts - especially coconut crab and giant clams.
- Coconut, island cabbage, manioc, yams, taro, banana, and other native fruits.

The most common trait these diets shared were based on whole, unrefined, nutrient-dense foods.

CHAPTER 8

Who Defines Food?

We refer to *food* as if it is a given: "This is what we eat and therefore this is food". *Food* is a nebulous idea, as much of what we eat is not, by strict definition, "food". For instance, an elk is a living creature. Yes, we hunt it, kill it, butcher it and dress it - all so that we can consume the animal - but is the living creature just that, or is it food? At some point, we evolved to recognize that we could use the elk as a food source, and the same could be said about the many other insects and animals we eat. So too do most plants have to be killed or wounded in order for us to use the consumable parts of the plant to supply the desirable nutrients we are seeking, and discard or properly prepare the parts of the plant that may have an abundance of undesirable toxins. There are many herbivores that eat large amounts of plant matter that we humans simply could not digest, and in some cases, could kill a human. Yet, to that herbivore, it is food. Getting food from our environment came about through many adaptations and evolutionary forces within our ecology. What I propose here is that the word food is something that *is meant to be* consumed, and the caveat is that living creatures can be, and are, consumed as food.

To the best of my knowledge, there are only a few substances in nature that are *meant to be* eaten, and therefore exist to be "food:" tree sap, fruit, honey, and milk. Aside from that, I am not aware of any other thing created by nature that is inherently created to be consumed. Which begs the question: Who defines food? My answer: the individual life form does. The individual and their particular biology define what food is to them. Food is something that is taken from the environment that supplies the nutrients needed, and is low in toxins. However, what can be eaten safely by one individual, could be detrimental to another. Just about anything that we eat can not be eaten by someone who has an intolerance or allergy preventing them from being able to experience it as food.

For the most part, rice can be considered a hypoallergenic food. There are billions of people on the continent of Asia that eat the grain every day, yet there are many people out there that have extreme rice intolerance. Many people eat large amounts of nuts and seeds, yet some could die from anaphylactic shock from just a tiny trace of nuts or seeds in their meal. Entire cultures subsist on shellfish, yet so many people suffer from shellfish allergy. Whether someone has an allergy to a food - or must avoid certain foods, as if avoiding the plague because it will bring about extreme gastrointestinal pain, or cause excessive gas, or raise their blood sugar, or the list goes on - let us acknowledge that food is what food is to that particular person.

The same goes for what constitutes what is healthy food - it's going to be healthy for the individual and for their context. I've met people who thrive as vegetarians, and I've met those who thrive as carnivores. People will argue and debate about which extreme is best for everyone, but in all honesty, the proof is in the pudding: people can thrive on either diet, whether each side likes it or not. It is laughable to me that someone who dies at the age of 70 will be attacked by an opposing food cult as proof that their diet failed them because that individual did not experience extreme longevity, in order to support their stance. This type of validation occurs all the time in the diet/health industry, and yet, they all seem to forget that nearly everyone who eats any diet will die. They seem to forget that healthy and robust people appear to die as well.

Excuse the sarcasm. The point is, food alone will not, and cannot, fix every biological reality we each face. Until a clan of immortals are discovered, we have to relate to food a little differently than what seems to be the norm. Extreme longevity is likely not going to be derived from food, and if immortality is what you are pursuing, then perhaps a deep study of alchemy will get you close. The idea that food is defined at large by outside authorities, and is imposed on us with particular expected results, is what I consider to be a sickness in our culture. It's monotheism applied to diet and it denies the inherent wildness of our bodies. Dietary wisdom can be found in a more polytheistic way of relating to the forces that govern the multiverse that is diet and nutrition. Nutrition can serve many purposes and I believe that quality of life is an important purpose for us to relate to diet.

Worshiping at the Altar of a Dietary God

Many people today worship at the altar of a dietary god. We see this in the way that popular diets have followings and cults similar in spirit to those of monotheistic religions. Diets like keto, carnivore, low-fat, paleo, veganism, vegetarianism, and so on, all reveal this type of landscape of view. It is understandable, as many humans find a lot of meaning and self-identity when having a secular relationship in organizing one's diet. Yet, if one spends any amount of serious time in different nutritional circles, it is likely to encounter people who will defend their way of eating at all costs. It is baffling that some will violently defend their diet, even if their health continues to fall apart while being on it. People preach to others, attack others with different viewpoints, rationalize their own reasoning, and will even lie in order to promote their particular dietary god. People get brainwashed, shamed, and punished for their perceived sins in these circles. Heaven forbid, a newbie on the Keto diet tells diehard Keto people that they ate a banana! That newbie will be onslaught with explanations that they have just invoked the plague onto all of humankind. I wish this was all hyperbole. This happens all the time! We exist in a monotheistic culture, and just as many have fought over the "one, true God", many are fighting over "the one, true diet." The arguments sound like this:

"This ______ diet is the best diet that has ever existed."
"True health can only be achieved through ______ diet."
"The other diets will make you sick."
"Everyone must have a high-carb and low-fat diet in order to lose weight."
"It is important that you are in ketosis all of the time and count every carbohydrate to ensure you are not kicked out of ketosis."
"Ignore the others; you must have high amounts of protein in your diet in order to get it right!"
"We are meant to eat a plant-based diet only."
"We are all carnivores and eating plants will hurt you".

You see the pattern? To put it in the most eloquent way possible - this is nonsense! Humans have existed, reproduced, and thrived long before the dietary gurus bottled up their sanitized ideas and shoved them down our throats. My goal here is to back away from these narrow concepts and promote a broader way of looking at the *human diet*, with some principles for narrowing it down to the individual, while reminding us that it may change drastically from year to year. I suggest that we all be open and receptive to the diversity possible with diet, for oneself and for others. The true way of ancestral nutrition is polytheistic.

CHAPTER 9

Healing a Fundamental Relationship

Ancestral nutrition is about transforming our entire relationship with food so that it becomes rewarding and nourishing - a form of conscious love. This is a process of learning to relate to food as nectar that bestows and supports a full life. For humans, the spoils of the hunt and the fruits of the land are like honey to the bee: innate and essential. Beyond our individual diet, there is an essence of an overarching drive towards life whenever we eat. This drive has been present since the beginning of life, where the first life forms were being guided by their mouths on the ocean floor. To live, we must consume. Yet, as we've explored a bit, it can be so much more than that. Food can bring groups of different people together for celebrations and festivities. Feeding those who are less fortunate can be a part of a spiritual pathway. Eating together can act as a glue, binding entire communities together, and sometimes bringing peace between enemies. We build cultures with food. Food can be holy and shared with the gods and with other spirits. It can be an anchor in time and space.

Without food, the potential of the human soul withers and fades. If one has never known true hunger in one's life, let us be grateful for that blessing! Rumi once remarked: "The satiated man and the hungry man do not see the same thing when they look upon a loaf of bread." Someone who feels satisfied and full is going to feel entirely differently than someone who feels deprived and empty. The options these different people have, and what they can contribute to, differ to a radical degree.

Eating food can be as comforting as a warm embrace or the tenderness of a loving hand. The potential for our relationship to food to be this nurturing starts when we are babies, suckling at the breasts of our mothers, grasping for the essence of life with our mouths. Yet, it is possible to have a full belly of high-quality food and still feel empty, undernourished, and deprived. Learning to be satisfied here is critical. If deep down in our psychosomatic processing of reality we feel our needs are not being met, and we are driven by a rabid longing to end the pain of feeling empty inside, then perhaps the best diet on earth will not help us. If we cannot reach out, take in, and receive nourishment, then we starve ourselves regardless of what we eat. Yet, for those who have felt true hunger, the drive to eat can push our behavior to the greatest of extremes. The impulse to feed the hungry mouths around us, can turn any decent human toward the depths of desperation where the lines of rules become blurred.

The primary essence of ancestral nutrition is nourishment. Not the appearance of it, but its actual existence. I believe that it is essential to be honest with ourselves around our relationship with food. Meditating on this can go a long way in supporting us in our process as we discover our innate motivations when it comes to any particular diet. If we do not know what those motivations are, we will likely create self-sabotaging behaviors that will interfere with our ability to heal and thrive. If we are not conscious of the choices we make when it comes to what we consume, a cascade of choices that will reach deep into our future may lead to inauspicious effects.

Thus far, we have reflected on the context of food and living creatures - the dance of life consuming life. Now we can start to explore what our ancestors can teach us about how we might go about relating to food in these modern times. Once again, The Way of Ancestral Nutrition does not seek to eat exactly like our ancestors did; but to take on the spirit of our ancestors when making decisions about what to consume in our current world-wide landscape, and to honor the very expression of the ancestors - in ourselves. These are the megaliths that we can lean on, or see in the distance to help us find our way.

Adaptability

Being adaptable is one of the hallmarks of what makes us human and also what makes us the most prolific species on the planet. Human beings can survive off a wide variety of foods and dietary configurations. With this, I suggest we call upon the spirit of adaptability for our dietary choices. If a diet is based solely off of a few foods that are restrictive for our budget, hard to find, difficult to manage when traveling or during high stress situations, the diet is likely to fail us because it does not possess the requisite adaptability to survive in the world as it is now. Allowing our diet to have elements which make it adaptable is absolutely key. The best way to do that is to allow yourself as broad a variety of foods as your body can tolerate, and to do your best not to live on highly restrictive diets, if possible. Now, some of us may require a restrictive diet to be healthy, and this is okay. I certainly have restrictions. To benefit from adaptability here, I suggest we invoke the power of "as broad as our body can tolerate." However, if you can, eat the rainbow, the sea, the grasslands, and the jungles in a manner that is as sustainable as you can afford.

A major element to consider with adaptability is developing the skill of eating on-the-go, and having different degrees of acceptability, while holding true to a thriving directive. Be not afraid to simply eat a whole block of cheese and an apple if that is what you have access to. Learn to be creative and make the most out of your environment and what is available within it. Personally, I will scale from whole fruit to juice as it is required. Foods with the least amount of processing and the most nutrients are my reference point in choosing what foods enter my body. With that, I can find acceptable meals in most places, and not feel deprived, even with my restrictions. In the name of adaptability, if all else fails, I am willing to fast until "real food" is available to me.

In regards to individual adaptability, the best diet for *you* is going to be the best diet for you at *that* given time and will provide the amount of nutrients that you need then. Be willing to accept that what works now may not work later, and begin the work again after you have completed the previous cycle. The body is wild! Be flexible, be attentive to your needs, and adjust as necessary. Learn to experiment and to not be afraid to try new configurations if your current results are not what you would like. The truest dietary authority you will ever encounter is the one that is within.

Within the scope of ancestral principles and the use of common sense, there is a wide range of possibilities. Be willing to listen to your body and see what type of feedback you get. Allow yourself to eat six meals one day and two the next if that is what is authentically being communicated. Trust in yourself. Avoid becoming rigid and mechanical. If you are feeling better, relying less on stimulants, feel calmer, have lasting energy, and see your libido increasing, then it is probably a good path for you. If you feel the opposite, then maybe not so much. Some may find multiple configurations give them the same results. In these cases, it will come down to personal preference. Listen to the wisdom of the body.

Adaptability also applies to how we distribute our food acquiring behaviors. I would recommend against going severely out of one's way in order to acquire a special vegetable or fruit that someone has deemed essential to health. If a food item is only available in a store that is two hours away, we may need to ask ourselves, "Is it worth it?" There is no single food that is essential to health. I would also advise against spending large amounts of money on something that is not going to have a significant energetic place in one's diet. For example, spending $40 on 4 ounces of wild organic acai berry, when one's food budget for the week is $120.00. Those resources could have been better spent on other, more important foods. Wouldn't you say? Lastly, shop within your budget; invest a *reasonable* amount of time in acquiring and preparing the food; and don't drown under massive waves of extra stress to create the most incredible diet ever composed. If one's lifestyle cannot support it, it is meaningless to become obsessive about making sure that a diet is composed of the most pristine and organic ingredients possible. Some extra stress is okay, and in some cases, probably necessary and worth it. We must weigh the cost-to-benefit ratio against the other factors in our lives when it comes to determining our diet.

Another thing to consider would be the lowest energy investment for the highest payoff. In a lifestyle where the acquisition of food-based energy is often energetically expensive and potentially dangerous, getting the highest return on investment is essential. A hunter-gatherer would not go over huge leaps and bounds for a poor energetic pay-off. Energy conservation is a hallmark of living creatures, and spending it often requires good reason. From an energetic standpoint, this also presents a strong case for why meat, fruits, and tubers are often more useful than vegetables. Meats, fruits, and tubers supply all the necessary nutrients we could ever need with a much more caloric energetic load. Vegetables may be useful for other reasons, of course, but not for energy. This realization can aid in adaptability if you can get creative. If you are on the run, need energy, and have to choose between a baked potato or a vegetable-only salad, it may be better to go with the potato.

Nutrient Density and Diversity

Universally, ancestral diets were nutrient dense. They were especially dense in micronutrients, as the ancestors' sources for carbohydrates, protein and fat would substantially fluctuate at various times. Our ancestors relied on whole, fresh, local, and unprocessed foods that were mined from the depths of nature. Nature still offers us a nutritious bounty, and having a diet that is jam-packed with a variety of nutrients is the key to a nourishing diet. We want a diet that promotes thriving, is robust, and is resistant to holes. Ideally, our diets would not be lacking in any of the essential nutrients. We want a diet that is providing enough vitamins, minerals, phytochemicals, zoochemicals, and macronutrients. While the Reference Daily Intake is a useful reference point, it has limited value because our unique bodies are the ultimate barometer for nutrient intake. Our individual, daily nutrient allowance is relative to our particular inheritances and our individual chosen ways of life.

If you have access, and the means to acquire it, making it a priority to supply yourself with an abundance of what the body needs is going to provide auspicious results. Over-nourish yourself with nutrient density! You *want* to create a state in which you cannot possibly improve your health any further by adding more nutrients. In this way, further increases in vitality are not dependent on diets, which have their limits. Of course, being replete with the various nutrients required by your body will not solve all of your woes in life, but it will go a long way toward removing a rate-limiting step. However, as much as we want to make sure our bodies are not needing anything, we want to ensure that we aren't taking in so many nutrients that our bodies begin to shift them into poisons.

Fortunately, we have access to some nutritional powerhouses in today's world, and I will list them next. There are a lot of highly nutritious foods that will not be listed, so please do not let this list limit you. The following just happen to be more easily attainable, accessible and economical:

Liver:

Liver contains large amounts of vitamins A (around 20,000 IU per 4 ounces), D, E, K, folic acid, copper, zinc, riboflavin, pyridoxine, B12, and carnitine.

All forms of liver are nutritious. However, eating too much liver from *ruminants* can be problematic. Liver from poultry may be the best option as it is lower in copper, yet sufficiently supplies vitamin A, and other energy nutrients. Copper is an essential nutrient and many of us can afford to eat a bit more of it. For these reasons, I eat 2-4 ounces of ruminant liver about twice a week, and other meals contain chicken liver.

Liver has been considered a sacred food in many cultures, and hunters all over the world have been known to eat the liver raw - right out of their kill. While I do not have that particular tradition in my own life, I do partake in the consumption of quite a bit of liver. I cycle off of it from time to time, depending on what my body is asking for, and I vary it up by consuming liver from lamb, beef, bison, and chicken. If you cannot stomach liver, supplementing with liver tablets may be useful. I recommend "Vital Proteins" as a liver supplement source.

Heart:
Heart supplies an abundance of B vitamins, zinc, and copper. It supplies several energy nutrients like Coenzyme Q10, an antioxidant involved in energy production.

Red meat:
Red meat is loaded with most of the B vitamins, zinc, and iron.

Eggs:
Eggs are one of nature's most perfect foods. They are jam-packed with nutrition; they contain vitamins A, D, E, K, B vitamins, selenium, and the building blocks of steroid synthesis cholesterol. However, one of the best nutritional qualities of eggs comes from its high amount of choline. For some of the most nutritionally dense eggs available on the market today, check out "Eggland's Best Cage-Free" eggs. Just compare their label to other eggs and you'll see what I mean. Local

eggs, or even eggs from your own chickens, are also great options if available.

Brazil nuts:
The biggest benefit of the Brazil nut is that it contains an abundance of selenium. They have a variety of other nutrients in small amounts.

Seaweed:
Seaweed is loaded with iodine and other trace minerals.

Molasses:
If you do not have blood sugar issues and tolerate sugars well, then molasses is quite nutritious. It is perhaps the best food source of potassium there is on a gram-for-gram basis. One tablespoon of good quality molasses offers 20% of the daily value of potassium. Most diets that do not supply an abundance of calories tend to severely lack potassium, and although many foods contain potassium, many do not supply enough of it overall.

Leafy greens (spinach, swiss chard, turnip greens, beet greens, collard greens, etc.):
Leafy greens rank high in potassium, iron, vitamin C, folate, K1, and calcium.

Bivalves (a.k.a oysters, clams, and mollusks):
Bivalves are extremely nutritious and are overall loaded with minerals like iron, zinc, copper, selenium, and manganese.

Potatoes:
Contrary to most popular food culture movements, potatoes are quite nutritious. They contain even more nutrients than the more popular sweet potato. They rank high in potassium, vitamin B6, vitamin C,

and manganese, and they also supply a good dose of many other necessary micronutrients.

Sweet potatoes:
Sweet potatoes are high in vitamin A, vitamin C, manganese, and potassium.

Avocados:
Avocados are high in potassium, vitamin E, vitamin K, B5, B6, copper, and folate.

Beets:
Red and gold beets are high in folate (vitamin B9), betaine, vitamin A, manganese, potassium, iron, and vitamin C.

Orange Juice:
If your body can handle liquid calories high in carbohydrate, then orange juice is jam-packed with nutrition. It is high in vitamin C, folate, potassium, thiamine, and magnesium. Useful for very active people in reasonable dosages. Fresh is always better than pre packaged,

A diverse diet offers a greater range of adaptability. Naturally, there are dietary staples, and it does appear that most traditional cultures had at least, one or two, somewhat consistent, food allies in their diets. We can certainly benefit from some staples in our diet; however, if you only have a small range of acceptable food on your list, as is common in restrictive or elimination diets, then your ability to travel, shop, or enjoy life may be limited. These diets can definitely play an important role at different times for different people when it comes to the healing process; but if you impose these restrictions on yourself without need, it may be useful to ask yourself why you're doing so.

A healthy ecosystem is diverse with a variety of different ferns and fauna. *You* are an ecosystem of cells, bacteria, viruses, and fungi. A diet that supplies a diverse amount of plant and animal nutrients is a nod to this instinctive need for variation. Hunter-gatherer tribes had access to a very wide array of plants and animals, and some still do. Even in the case of eating a whole carcass, the variety of organs, different cuts of meat, and different bones is quite high. It is a good idea to rotate out the different plants and animals you're eating to some degree, so that your food ecosystem can shift and cycle as it needs. Do remember to balance this with your energetic investments as well.

"Poison is in everything, and no thing is without poison. The dosage makes it either a poison or a remedy." - Paracelsus

A diverse diet not only has a better chance at casting a holistic net of the required nutrients; it can also keep plant toxins low by preventing toxins that naturally occur in plants from oversaturating our pathways. To discuss the topic of nutrient density, we are required to dance with the subject of toxins. Natural toxin exposure is a given, and these days, so are human-made toxins. Ancestral diets were low in toxins and were high in nutrients - the definition of a high quality diet. All plants contain toxins, many of which we call antioxidants, meant to protect them from fungi, bacterial infections, insects, and other threats. However, those antioxidants are not there to protect *us*; they are present to protect the plants. Our physiology has evolved with many plant toxins over eons and has learned to process them in beneficial ways. As we consume the antioxidants, our bodies have a cellular stress response to them and exorcise them. In the process of exorcism, certain pathways work vigorously, and by default, become stronger - hence the message that antioxidants are good for us.

Everything that is alive has an impulse and biological imperative to protect itself. It does not seem that most living things want to willingly hand over their personhood to another species to be consumed. In the same vein, most species must devour another in order to live. So how does nature deal with these seemingly antagonistic agendas? Species develop a strategy of defense. It can be a strategy to fight, flee, deflect, or block. The strategies are diverse, such as injecting sharp quills into an attacker, or spraying liquid while fleeing, or even fighting and injecting poison. Animals tend to defend themselves in kinetic ways, and plants tend to weaponize their inherent toxic elements.

Plants are no exception to the apparent rule of having a biological impulse to protect themselves. They too are alive and do not *want* to be eaten. As much as some nutritional circles claim that plants are willing participants in this dance of life and death - of eat or be eaten - plants do not appear to be as willing, as it turns out that all plants develop defenses to ward off those who would freely eat them. We can find that many of the plants we eat have defenses. The fruits and vegetables most common in our food supply tend to deploy mild, relatively benign, toxins. The reproductive parts of plants, like legumes, nuts, seeds, and especially grains tend to work with a more noxious type of weaponry, because if they are over-consumed the species dies. Traditional cultures took great care in preparing foods like legumes and grains with methods that reduced the toxin load. This included soaking, sprouting, and fermenting them. They avoided certain poisonous plants, or cooked certain, potentially poisonous or highly toxic plants to inhibit the effect of the plant toxin on the human. Eating these foods without conscious deliberation of their potential dangers was unwise. Today's modern farming methods have only concentrated the toxins of many plant foods we eat.

Overall, at this stage in our evolutionary history, the mixing of gene pools and the pressures exerted on our genome over generations have given us a broad mix of what people are capable of digesting and absorbing. The key here is to understand general principles, and to know how *your* own body responds to different toxins. In most cases, the severity of a food toxin is dependent on who is consuming it. If you can eat grains and legumes, and do not suffer ill consequences, such as reduced health, indigestion, or inflammation, then perhaps your ancestry favors these foods. In general, it is probably best to lean toward traditional preparation methods for foods like grains and legumes. Nowadays, we also have to be prepared to defend against man-made toxins in our food supply, and therefore, sourcing organic, local food, or even growing our own organic foods, may be wise. I also recommend we all do our best to keep an eye on food recall lists. Having a high ratio of beneficial nutrients to toxins is a pillar of any ancestral diet.

Eat As Often As You Must & Eat As Infrequently As Possible

Our ancestors were not necessarily having three square meals a day, and it was not uncommon to have small windows of food scarcity. They did not have refrigerators, or cardboard boxes full of food that were readily available. They also did not have constant demands on their time, chronic stresses, performance metrics, artificial toxin exposure, and the same health challenges many of us do now. They had more downtime and were capable of being "less productive" much of the time. So meal frequency is a situation in which we can take cues from our ancestors, which we must balance against pragmatic reality.

When we do not eat, or rather, when we fast, we are undergoing a type of stress. Not all stressors are negative and fasting can have a wide variety of health benefits if you can deal with its impact holistically. In fact, fasting has a long history of use in many cultures, and often occurs naturally in humans who dwell in wild places and eat from the land. However, we must acknowledge that fasting works for some people, and does not work for everyone. I find that a lot of people who are deeply stressed out tend to gravitate toward fasting, because it adds to the momentum that they have already created – a biological paradigm of stress. If fasting begins to lead to erosion of certain parts of the body though, it has little value. I would suggest that anyone who has a very fast-paced and hectic schedule, or has a constitution that may be on the weaker side, to be gentle with fasting.

As I've mentioned, food fortifies our being, but it can also clog certain pathways at times. The body is designed to go periods without eating, yet, we must find natural ways to fast if we are to do it consistently. Skipping breakfast or dinner on some days may be all that is accessible and healthy for some. If you are not feeling particularly hungry, then I would not try to force a meal at that time. If you are feeling especially hungry, then by all means, eat! I encourage you to be organic with the process of intermittent fasting. Longer fasts can have some therapeutic value, but how to go about those types of fasts is beyond the scope of this work, so I highly recommend seeking trusted counsel on this if you are interested in the subject.

As for meal frequency in general, I believe this can also have an organic flow. Eat as often as you must and eat as infrequently as possible. This may change from day to day, or period to period. Real hunger is a call to eat. If you are busy, charging along at full throttle and at the edge of your capacity, your meal frequency may look like six meals a day. Other days, or during slower periods that do not require you to be at your edge, you may have two meals a day. Free yourself from the notion that you must always eat one particular way forever. If you are fasting and your health, energy, vitality, and lust for life are increasing, or at least being supported, then you're probably heading in the right direction. If they are not, and all of these areas have you feeling like you are backsliding, you may need to readjust something. You may need to titrate the periods where you have more meals and times where you have less meals - it's all going to depend on what you need at that time. The healthier you become, the less you may need to eat. The more health problems and overall stress you face - whether it's positive or negative stress for that matter - the more you may need to eat. By extension, this same principle applies to how much to eat as well: eat as little as you can, and eat as much as necessary. If nourishing oneself to support thriving is the food culture, then overeating and undereating are both undesirable, but it's also contextual. It all depends on the circumstances that you are facing at any particular time.

For those who are merely interested in fasting for fat loss, I feel it important to note that the fat on your body is not just a dormant, sluggish, inert substance. Fat can be considered both an endocrine gland and a toxin disposal site. Body fat releases, increases, and modifies a variety of hormones. Due to its insulating nature, fat supplies a safe place to store toxins, especially man-made toxins. Put simply, body fat does serve a larger purpose. When we begin to lose large amounts of fat, it will undoubtedly change our inner experience of ourselves, but on deeper levels than just emotional or confidence levels. The more fat one loses, the more drastic the inner, chemical landscape must change and shift. The body will temporarily contend with a toxin dump, which can make it difficult and demanding on the resources it has. In a lot of ways, I find that focusing the lens on fat loss is not always the best focus to have. Instead, if we build up our inner resources with nutritious food; move in ways that feed our bodies and minds; and release our attachment to protective barriers, that express as excessive layers of fat (relative to the individual) that create a shield to our muscular core, we may find that fat dissolves off the frame organically. This is not to say this will happen for everyone. You alone will need to determine how you approach your frame of focus. In the end, I suggest that you become at least tangentially familiar with functional forms of eating as a useful skill set. The Way of Ancestral Nutrition is concerned with thriving - the rest is outside of the scope of this work.

Fear Not the Unknown

In many nutritional circles, there is so much fear around eating in ways that fall outside of conventional formats. Some nutritionists may shriek in horror at the thought of humans eating only meat and shunning vegetables. Yet humans do it, and have done it, to no drastic ill effect for eons. There are tribes in the Amazon who shun pure water in their daily lives and only drink spit beer and tea. We humans are resilient creatures. I am not saying that we should ignore, or not take advantage of, scientific inquiry, for the ability to take ideas and test them in rigorous ways is certainly a useful tool. Let us not forget though, that humans have survived and thrived on this planet long before the notion of science existed.

Many hunter-gatherers of the present are robust, vital, happy people that eat from what is available to them in nature. Some are predominantly carnivorous, eating very little plant matter, whereas others eat mostly what they can gather, and many fall somewhere in between. They are not counting calories and obsessing over macronutrient ratios. They do not wait for messengers to share with them the latest study about how meat is going to kill them or how special berries will help them live longer. I am not suggesting that we simply imitate this "free-form" way of eating, although one could if they wanted to. I state this to help us free ourselves from the mental traps that we find ourselves in around food in these modern times, where fear and our desire to control every aspect of our existence is reflected in our food culture.

Relying on the simplicity of natural foods from multiple classes, understanding the inherent adaptability of humans, and listening to our wild bodies is going to provide a solid and stable bedrock in the constantly changing winds of nutrition. With that stability in mind, and an understanding of our hunter-gather heritage, we can then study the science, experiment, get biofeedback, and adjust based on our unique genetic and health circumstances. Your diet may not look like anything currently recommended, and yet be ideal for you. Fear not the unknown.

CHAPTER 10

Rewilding Through Conscious Food Choices

"To bring wild animals under the control of humans over a long period of time for the purpose of providing useful products and services; the process involves careful handling, breeding, and care. If humans cannot control and modify an animal's appearance or behavior, the animal is not fully domesticated."
- from the Curriculum for Agriculture Science Education

Rewilding is a possibility only when something has ceased to be wild. As humans, we pursue rewilding based on the understanding that we are currently a domesticated phenotype of Homo sapiens, and that reigniting the wildness inside of us has special gifts that can deeply enrich our lives. The essence of domestication is control - control over food, sexuality, shelter, schedule, appearance, and temperament. Indeed, to be free to choose is a wild trait. To be honest though, the term rewilding seems like yet another nebulous term. I think that what rewilding actually means to humans living in an industrial, commodified, computerized society such as ours - which seems to intend on remaining so - is open for interpretation. Some of these interpretations are quite literal, with a focus on outdoor movement, bush craft disciplines, and simpler living, while others can be more internalized and concerned with the essence of who we are. To my understanding, the one element common to all interpretations, is the casting off of the shackles binding us to conditioned ways of being that are not freely chosen. To be wild is to lead a more sovereign existence - it is liberation.

Regardless of where you find yourself, resisting the domesticating force with a wild inner state is possible. Rewilding is not just a way to engage in the literal hunter-gatherer patterns of behavior; rewilding is an awakening of a state in which we are self-directed, self-willed, conscious creatures, as free as we can be. There is a mechanical, self-perpetuating monster devouring the human spirit. It locks up our movement capacity in a cage shaped like a cubicle; it neuters our expressive sexuality with perverted morality; it reduces our vital spirit with denatured food; and then picks its teeth with bones from our ancestral history. To rewild is to regenerate lost parts of ourselves.

To me, the truest essence of being wild is to be self-possessed. This is the most beautiful and sacred lesson I learned from working at the wolf sanctuary. Domesticated animals are asleep to their true capacity for self-possession, for they live under the rules of masters and shepherds. If they do not comply, then they are cast aside, abandoned, or killed. Obedience ensures temporary survival. They are not meant to think for themselves or be especially self-possessed. They are not meant to question the walls of their existence. Beginning the process of rewilding requires us to take individual steps towards loosening the bindings on us; and one of the simplest, most accessible ways to begin is by becoming conscious of what we are eating.

One of the elements of our domestication is to have our food choices controlled. In a lot of ways, we are like cattle - being told what to eat, on what patch of grass we can roam, and when to come back into the barn. If our relationship to food is being exploited by commercialization, careful marketing, propaganda, food authorities, or government institutions, then there inherently exists a layer of control. Taking back our food choices under our own authority is one of the most accessible ways we can begin to rewild and we can begin to do so today. Here are some basic steps that can assist you in your rewilding process with food.

1. Become Conscious.

Wake up and become aware of this ancient, dynamic process of consuming the world around you, in order to live. So long as you are alive, you will exist within this drama. What are the variables? What are you eating? Where was it made? Who was it made by and what are the company's practices?

2. Educate yourself.

Begin to learn about nutrition for yourself, and do not take anyone's word for what you should and should not be eating. Use common sense, read books, watch videos, consult specialists, and get different opinions. Study high-fat, low-fat, vegetarian, vegan, carnivore diets, and everything in between. This is so you can understand the territory you roam; determine what is edible and what is poisonous; and to not blindly follow others.

3. Experiment.

Ultimately, you are the best resource for what works best, because it is your unique, organic existence which you are seeking to nourish and sustain. Test your ideas on yourself, and listen to your body.

4. Refine.
This is a lifelong, ever-evolving process of balancing your body's needs, getting better, and adjusting what you are eating based on how your body changes and what becomes available.

Your internal landscape is your domain. Since you are human, you are the greatest and most adaptable food acquirer in known history. If you choose, you can take control of your own food by growing your own food, stewarding your own food, and by hunting for your own food. If you have the means to do so, by all means, please do! However, the sad reality is that this may not be accessible to all of us. The spirit of owning our relationship to food is accessible to those of us who are fortunate enough to exist in a country with a reasonable degree of resources available to do so. Those of us who can't grow, shepherd or hunt for our food on plots of land, can make use of our carefully sharpened mental and emotional tools, and hunt and gather in our supermarkets.

A Framework for Transitioning to a Type of Ancestral Diet

Based on everything communicated thus far, I hope I have been able to transmit the falsity that there is any one dietary configuration that could be representative of the ancestral. For those of you who may have wanted a framework for adopting a way of eating a diet that is more "ancestral-like" so to speak, I hope that the following can serve as a basic platform for you to use in our modern world. Although I have my own suggestions, these are not to be mistaken as official dietary recommendations. Consider them to be like a midwife, helping you to birth a new process in your relationship with food. As with most diets, it may not be a platform that works for all.

Week One:

- **Remove sugary drinks and drink water, coffee, and tea only.** If you are very active, fruit juice can be added in small amounts. Eight cups of water, or tea, per day is a good starting point, but adjust as needed based on your own thirst signals.
- **Add color to all of your meals.** Prioritize having more color on your plate by adding foods like leafy greens, dark red tomatoes, fresh green herbs, different types and colored spices, multi-colored carrots, and so on.
- **Eat high protein foods at least twice a day.** If you are not committed to being a vegetarian or vegan, animal protein is ideal. If you are not used to eating animal protein multiple times a day, start by introducing a little fish, plain chicken, a couple of eggs, or by adding gelatin to some of your meals, little by little. These proteins tend to be easier to digest than muscle meat. Your digestion may need to adjust to the increased animal protein and you may feel uncomfortable *initially*; it should not be a permanent fixture.
- **Right from the start, remove the use of all industrial oils such as: corn, canola, soy, grapeseed, and anything labeled as vegetable oil.** These oils are all very high in oxidized and inflammatory fats; also, they have only existed a few decades. Swap them out with butter, coconut oil, tallow, olive oil, and other animal fats instead.

Week Two:

- **Begin the process of removing most grains from your diet.** This may not need to be permanent, but stop consuming them for a period of three months, at least. Then, if you want to, reintroduce gluten-free grains (like corn, certified gluten-free oats, rice, etc.) and/or sprouted, gluten-containing grains thereafter. The key here is to see what happens when you reintroduce the grain back into your diet. How is your digestion, your energy, and your mood after you eat them again? If any of these areas take any type of hit, avoid that particular grain, or grains in general. Some people tolerate them, and do just fine, yet many do not. I cannot tolerate grains at all, whereas my wife seems to do fine with them on occasion.
- **Replace grains with starches** such as potatoes, sweet potatoes, taro, plantains, yuca/cassava/tapioca, turnips, and parsnips.
- **Slowly begin to add other healthy fats to your meals**, such as one to two tablespoons of red palm kernel oil, ghee, or avocado oil, as well as include more actual avocados into your diet. Your gallbladder may need to adjust to the increased fat intake, so pay attention to your digestion as you introduce more fat to your meals.
- **If your digestion is doing well with the increase in protein in your daily meals, and you are enjoying the animal protein, experiment with having protein present at most of your meals for a while.** You may get to the point where your hunger may dictate a different avenue, but learning true hunger signals takes time.

- **Start the process of cutting out all forms of sugar - even the sugar substitutes.** Begin to add more fruit to your diet. If you struggle with this one, try eating a small amount of 75% or above, dark chocolate to feed the sweet tooth, or use natural sweeteners like honey, molasses, or maple syrup to lightly sweeten your meals or snacks. These natural sweeteners have nutrients in them and can be helpful when cutting out refined sugars from our diet. This one can be a rough transition for some people, but it is well worth it. Generally, refined sugar is negative for most people.

Third Week

- **Try removing legumes, including soy, from your diet completely, or try only eating sprouted legumes.** For most people, legumes can be hard to digest and they have other compounds that can be difficult to tolerate. Treat them as you would grains for the most part. Consider eliminating them, reintroducing, observing, and then preferring the sprouted variety if you can tolerate them. Sprouted legumes are easy to find on Amazon and/or you can sprout your own.
- **Try removing natural sweeteners from your diet completely, or only eating them directly after intense exercise.** Consuming natural sugars after intense exercise increases your capacity to absorb carbs and helps prevent the sugar from becoming unhealthy.
- **Try cutting out dairy for a bit and evaluate.** Go a month without cheese, milk, and yogurt, and then reintroduce them and see what happens. If you experience no uncomfortable symptoms or a drop in energy, then perhaps you can keep them

in your diet. Dairy is very nutritious and packed full of beneficial compounds if you can tolerate it. I tend to prefer goat and sheep dairy over cow, but that is not a hard and fast rule.

<u>**Fourth Week**</u>

- **Begin to explore a larger variety of animal foods such as red meat and even organs!** Start adding a variety of shellfish as well, such as shrimp, oysters, and clams. It is best to add shellfish from reputable and sustainable-practices companies. Liver and heart are especially nutritious foods and can be wonderful for you. There are many recipes online that can make any organ taste delicious, and hide the fact that you are even eating them. You could also purchase organ sausages from "Grassland Beef" - they do not taste like organs and pack a nutritional punch.
- **Explore a larger variety of vegetables**, but do your best not to go crazy here. An excess of vegetables can be hard on some people's digestion, so start slow and find a comfortable place for you.
- **Try adding some nuts and seeds to your diet.** Do not overdo it though! Nuts and seeds can be easy to overeat, can be hard on digestion, are high in omega-6s, and can have some antinutrients in them. A small handful a day is not excessive. Like legumes, sprouted nuts and seeds are a lot easier for the human animal to digest.

There you have it: a straightforward and simple format for adopting an ancestral diet. This is only a starting point with a very basic profile. It may look completely different to you once you really dial it in over months and years of experimentation. You may find that a plant-based diet serves you better. You may find you need to cut out all starches, or sugars, or both. You may find you are best served as a carnivore. Consider the above a basic guideline and not a prescription.

At this point, the right type of diet for you is going to need to emerge out of self-discovery and experimentation. Regardless of how poor your current nutritional relationship may be, you can start making small changes towards healing that relationship, and eating a nutritious and wholesome diet today. For some of us, the thought of completely revamping our current diet may seem daunting, or even impossible; for others, a complete overhaul may feel like a real and immediate responsibility. The key is to start off where you are currently at, and to view it as a dynamic process. You do not need perfection right now, and you can work towards refinement as time goes on. It may not be easy, but the transition and refinement process can be simple.

ANCESTRAL CONSCIOUSNESS

"*Life can only be understood backwards, but it must be lived forwards.*" ~ Soren Kierkegaard

All of the various perspectives, practices and exercises, and elements of behavioral patterns brought into the fold of this work culminate with one objective behind it: the activation of a deeper, ancestrally resonant bandwidth of consciousness. The concept that defines Ancestral Now is, that by inhabiting this way of being, we can ignite various experiential changes that promote sovereignty and rootedness, as well as a sense of belonging to a current so broad and so deep, that we are both humbled and empowered by it. This humility and power can crack us open so that our hearts may be touched by both the beauty and the pain of the world. If we can do all of this, we can begin to create real change that will reverberate through time. I apprehend it to be a liberating force to feel and know ourselves as homegrown humans that do what human beings do, without the perverting influence of modern society, religion, politics, corrosive culture, and nefarious forces actively seeking to suppress our freedom.

One of the many gifts of the bandwidths of ancestral consciousness is a more immediate sense of primal and primordial forces. For those who desire it, it can also act as a platform for transpersonal expanded states of awareness. This portion of Ancestral Now asks us to step out of the daylight, and to set aside what the rational mind thinks and schemes about, so that we may let go of the illusion of certainty. If we accept this, we move into darker, perhaps murky, and mysterious territory now. Here, the wind howls eerily and the hair on the backs of our necks prickles as we enter into the world of animism, cosmic forces, magic, death, spirits, and the realm of the invisible. We will eventually return to the daylight, but for now, let us consciously set it aside.

Our ancestors lived in worlds that were dynamically alive, across multiple dimensions. They recognized that perhaps the world of the five senses was *not* total. Some might even say, when the whole of inherited myths and stories are accepted, that the world we know is a subset of an unseen one - that the unseen world is more real than this one. While sensory experience does a relatively fine job of helping us navigate, it does little to define the cosmic totality of existence.

The civilizing current has progressively sanitized our world of mystery and magic. It makes no apologies for this, and in fact, wears it as a badge of honor. "The lowly savages that came before us had it all wrong; and the ability to control nature is proof of our superiority!", is the broadcast that echoes out. There is complete arrogance in the assumption that all the humans that have come before us, and even many today who understand that the world is "haunted", have all been wrong. This, by default, claims that only one, very young, culture is correct: the western culture. The primary way this has been accomplished is not so much through "reason" (the proposed ethos of western materialistic science) but through the removal of consciousness from the world. Consciousness is no longer *within* nature, and neither is *our* consciousness a *part* of nature. This "reasoning" is what could be argued to be quite unreasonable.

Nonetheless, there are ways of knowing that go beyond reason and depend on direct, immersive experiences. The ancestral worldview is available for us to engage with, *if* we are willing to have an authentic expression of it born from our *current* experience. This is where we truly begin to immerse ourselves in the world once again.

CHAPTER 11

Animism - The Foundation of our Ancestral Worldview

"Colonial anthropologists in the 19th century coined the term 'animism' to explain the worldview they found literally everywhere, and then categorized it as a primitive 'mistake.' Yet for 98% of human history, 99.9% of our ancestors lived, breathed, and interacted with a world that they saw and felt to be animate — a world imbued with lifeforce and inhabited by and permeated with forces, with which we exist in ongoing relation. This animate vision was the water in which we swam, it was consciousness in its natural dwelling place, the normative way of seeing the world and our place in it. It wasn't a theory, a philosophy, or an idea. It wasn't, actually, an 'ism'. It was the felt experience of how things were. Which is why it has been commonly understood across the entire world for all of time, so inherent that in most cultures there wasn't even a word for it." - Joshua Michael Schrei of The Green Emerald Podcast

Animism essentially means that we experience - as opposed to intellectualize - the universe and everything in it, as animate and imbued with consciousness. The world for an animist is alive and pulsating with an ineffable breath of life. The trees, the stars, the lakes, rivers, oceans, and stones *are living.* This view is also extended to human-made objects such as walls, carpets, training tools, homes, and cars - though, perhaps, there is a difference in their quality. For the animist, there is a fundamental *essence* in existence.

One of my favorite "animist thinkers" is Joshua Michael Schrei, founder of "The Emerald" podcast. His assertion of our animistic roots is expressed by referring to it as "normative consciousness" - meaning that it is the normal baseline state of functioning for the human animal; it is innate. This statement stands on some rather giant shoulders when realizing that 99.9% of our ancestors, through the entire Paleolithic era, were animists. We emerged from a lineage spanning hundreds of thousands of years, if not more, wherein our ancestors inhabited this worldview from the world over.

Western culture, with a lineage of a couple thousand years, asserts itself in opposition to this heritage. Much of this has to do with definitions of personhood; the boundaries of what we call the living; and the concept of a clear, distinguishing line between self and non-self; between what is inside and what is outside. We live in a western cultural story, reinforced only by select groups of scientists with the loudest microphones, that tells us that there are clear boundaries between self, other, animated, and inanimate. In actuality, *this* is just an idea - a model - and is by no means an inarguable truth. It is just a story of materialism and separation. In some senses, this model of viewing the world could be considered modern day metaphysics.

Since this book is being written for a primarily western audience, it would feel incomplete to simply move forward without at least attempting to weaken the hold our inanimate, disenchanted worldview has on us. In some ways, animism still exists in cultures at war with it. You can see animism living in tattoo shops; gatherings of Dungeons & Dragons; in our favorite mascots; in corporate symbols; fetishes or charms; comic books; and many more contemporary cultural expressions. To an animist, words, ideas, and concepts can *be alive or possess power.* The animist view echoes from the past into these places, and there is a profound lingering within us for this way of interacting with the world.

I *could* try and make a case for animism, but I will not; for animism is best understood when it becomes a way of being, knowing, and engaging with the world. To even begin to understand animism, we must live like animists. To live like an animist is to live as humans evolved to. No, I will not argue for animism. Instead, I prefer to simply instill doubt in the contemporary worldview and loosen the coil. From there, I will offer ways to experience animism for yourself through animist practices. Practicing animism is useful, but working with practices that can only exist in an animist universe can be even better.

I will forewarn that the following section will propose more questions than answers. This was done with purpose, as the state of *not* knowing is fertile ground where magic can happen. For those who may have it, it may be useful to withhold your disbelief - just long enough to potentially be surprised.

Questions to Loosen The Coil

> *"You make the grass green. You make your highs and you make your lows. But you don't make it alone. You are making it out of your union with the universe. And so everything is a coincidence of contraries, a coincidence of you being there, and*

the universe being there. And everything is one at the same time, because there's no green without the grass and there's no green without you. So the greenness is a transaction that ties you and the grass together." - Robert Anton Wilson

What could be said to be yours? Is it your thoughts, your emotions, your body? What *actually* distinguishes you as separate and unique?

These liminal questions require us to acknowledge that we are a crossroads; a system of interconnecting relationships. We are a *process* and not a noun. Our bodies are not created by us; our bodies are an inheritance from ancestral forces. The bones within us come from minerals that were sequestered from the oceans, and they are now replenished by the foods we eat. The food we eat acquires their minerals from digested plants and/or from the soil they spring from. The soil in and of itself is a community of sunlight, microbes, decaying matter, water, and cycles of time. Plants connect into this matrix, and the animals we eat, eat the plants. The water inside of us comes from the oceans, rivers, lakes, and the rain; and that water is excreted in the form of our urine, sweat, or tears. It evaporates, condenses, and is always becoming. Where do the cycles of our bodies' water begin and end? The air we breathe is exhaled by trees, and the air we release is in turn, breathed by trees. Without this air, we could not think, feel, or act. We are cultivated and birthed out of starlight. The sun infuses us with light, and the body stores that light and is animated by it. This light from within urges us to rise and to act.

Contemplate what the impact the following has on you:
The food you eat; the practices you perform; the work that you do; the people you interact with; the media you take in; the place you live in; the amount of sleep you got last night; the spirits you pray or talk to. Reflect on the can of worms that *is* your entire lived history, and its impact on how you **feel right now**. Why do you feel the way you do at *this* moment?

Let us ponder on language itself!
Consider how words, ideas, and concepts shape the world and shape us. Think about how *we* shape words, ideas, and concepts as well. Consider how most thoughts are language based. Thoughtforms can be so powerful that certain thoughts have empowered humans to transform this planet. Do our minds use words, or do words use our minds?

Language - a vehicle through which we can think, was not created by those of us living today. In most cases, it was created by others over many generations. Even still, language is chopped up, remixed, and cooked into our thought streams. Essentially, language is reproduced by us, and it depends on our thinking and our speaking of it, to be kept alive.

Get curious with the reality of being largely circumstantial:
The culture you were born in, the time and place of your birth, the family you inherited, the economical situation you were raised in, the neighbors in your area that became friends, the languages you orient with, and the ancestral body you have, are all circumstances which have shaped who you are. The same is true for every other human going as

far back as we can imagine. To what degree do your actions distinctly spring from you?

Personhood:

Can you see, know, feel, or sense the reality that much of you is a relational, ever changing set of interactions? In which case, how do *you* define personhood? Why do you have certain criteria for it? Who gave you that criteria for personhood? Can you say with certainty that you have personhood? If personhood does exist, perhaps it resides in your raw consciousness. In that case, would it be useful to contemplate the boundaries of consciousness?

Walking the Animist Walk:

This exercise was originally shared with me by a friend who is a senior sorcerer and longtime occultist. His inspiration for this particular exercise is credited to David Abrams, author of "The Spell of the Sensuous", as he adapted it from his work and modified it for his purposes.

Take a walk in a wild place. The further off the beaten track, the better.
With each step, notice how it feels to push down into the ground.
Notice the sensations. Pay attention to where each step begins and ends.
Go deeper - sensation does not stop at the surface; it is inside the skin and it goes beyond it as well.
Notice that just as you are pushing down into the ground, the ground is pushing back up into you, holding you up. You may begin to feel lighter as you become more and more aware of the ground pushing up against you.

Now, notice that this interpenetrating sensation is not just limited to the ground.

Sense the air around you. Breathe it in, feel it on your skin. Notice the sensation of air just inside your skin, as well as beyond it. Air is in every cell wall; it's in every part of you.

Pay attention to the contrasting sensations of being pushed by and pushing against, extending outward to every object in your field of awareness; to every plant, to every animal.

As you become aware of this field of awareness, you may sense that it is aware of you - interpenetrating and intersubjective. If you can notice the presence of a tree, the tree can notice you.

Notice how when you become aware of sensations between you and the other, that it lacks true edges or boundaries. Let the perceived edges of you and the other blur.

Extend your awareness out into that field, and allow the field to extend within you. Extensional and intensional awareness bleeding into a single field of awareness.

At this point, you may get the feeling that you are really sensing the world as it truly is for the very first time.

This type of interaction with the environment is where we can begin to explore the world in a way that is immersive and relationship-based. In my experience, immersion, consciousness and relationship are at the root of animism. You are immersed in the world and it is immersed in you. All forces, objects, and subjects extend into and are part of one another. You are alive; the world is alive. If relational immersion is at the root of animism, consciousness itself is at the core. To an animist, matter is just another form of conscious experience. To an animist, some of the most profound lessons can be transmitted by animals, plants, stones, stars, planetary bodies, and other natural forces.

As has been throughout this book, my encouragement here is to find the innate and engage with ways to activate those streams of power. Animism is there, within you, ready to emerge; ancient and present, yet, perhaps in some senses, asleep. This section of Ancestral Consciousness will feed off of an animist view of the world - even if its overt mention begins to fall to the background, where in some senses it belongs - for as Joshua Michael Schrei has said in his own words, in indigenous cultures there was no "ism" for this way of viewing the world; only our normal consciousness. May we be like fish in water, swimming in an animist ocean.

Technologies of Consciousness

"Many scientific disciplines begin by not observing any sort of vital spark or consciousness in material events and proceed to deny that these things exist in living things, including themselves. Because consciousness does not fit into their mechanistic schemes they declare it illusory. Magicians make exactly the reverse argument. Observing consciousness in themselves and animals, they are magnanimous enough to extend it to all things to some degree—trees, amulets, planetary bodies, and all. This is a far more respectful and generous attitude than that of religions, most of whom won't even give animals a soul." -Peter J. Carroll, in "Liber Null and Psychonaut: An Introduction to Chaos Magic"

For any honest student of ancient, and/or indigenous, cultures, a stark truth shines forth like a giant watchtower in the night: they understand the primacy of consciousness. It becomes obvious when we see how much focus was placed on developing technologies that revolved around altering, manipulating, refining, or expressing consciousness. By technology, I do not mean a physical piece of machinery; but a set of tools applied to some aspect of existence or self, with the intent of accomplishing a relatively predictable outcome. Meditation, for example, is a meta-technology of consciousness with individual applications being micro level applications of it. Ritual is another form of meta-technology.

We can look at surviving traditions that have a long history to get a sense of what ancestral communities were practicing deep into the past, even though we have no way of knowing what precisely was being done. Based on what we do know, it appears that there is very little question that Paleolithic humans were engaging in some form of ritual, divine communion, magic, and ancestral veneration. This appears to have been related to hunting, gathering, combat, healing, working with the dead, navigating the underworld, and who knows what else. We also know that many of the ancestors engaged with some form of psychedelic, and/or mind-altering substances, including alcohol. It does not have to be a stretch of the imagination to envision the ritual use of mind-altering plants paired with primal music, orgies, dance, dressing in costumes, and communing with the dead or other powerful spirits, as commonplace. To one degree or another, all of these elements of ritual have existed in early polytheistic traditions, and have survived into some indigenous cultures present now. They possess viable, biological reasoning behind their uses. These rituals either took place under an open sky or in circular womb-like structures built into the earth. I will share my personal experience with some of these ancient and surviving technologies.

Before we dive into these technologies, it is important for me to address what people collectively call "shamanism" in the West. Shamanism is at the root of human spiritual traditions, for we know, with very little doubt, that tribal cultures the world over develop "shamans", and that tribes are at the root of humanity. Shamanism is a word with many issues and failings - the least of which is that it refers to the medicine-people of one particular tribe in Siberia - and has been co-opted to refer to all medicine-people. A bunch of contemporary forms of shamanism have sprouted, and while I'm sure they are well-meaning circles, they often fall extremely short in terms of power, efficacy, and in depth. I am just going to glide around that rabbit hole; however, the word does confer some utility in the case of this section, because it allows me to refer to a set of practices that we can all relate to at a basic level. In some senses, what this section points to, is what many of us in the West think of as shamanism.

A very straightforward example, of what I mean by technology of consciousness, is a sweat lodge. I had the privilege of partaking in a few sweat lodge ceremonies, held by a man with a legitimate lineage to traditional, Lakota medicine-peoples. It was, and has been, one of the most beautiful experiences I have ever had. We sat in a womb made of earthen materials, in pitch darkness except for the glow of ruby-red lava rocks that had been heated in a fire outside. The rocks glowed with a magnetic presence at the center of the dome structure. We all entered wearing minimal clothing, and we felt the earth firmly beneath us. The man guiding the process drummed, sang songs, and called on the spirits of the land and the ancestors of his spiritual lineage. As far as I could tell, they responded. Steam and heat poured into us, and purified our bodies through sweat; our breathing deepened as a result. I truly felt a deeper connection to the earth than at any other point in time before that. I felt elated; refreshed; touched. *This* is a technology of consciousness; a gift from an older time - a treasure from the ancestors.

Through the magical, mystical, and wisdom schools present today, we can see teachings that survived from Paleolithic and early Neolithic times. We see them in the birthplaces of the I-Ching, Tantra, meditation, alchemy, indigenous magic, and much more. Ritualistic, magical, and mystical practices are part of, and deeply rooted in, the human experience.

Indigenous Technologies of Consciousness in Action

One of the oldest traditions born from the late Paleolithic era has actually played a large part in my understanding of this. I grew up in a tradition that has its roots in West Africa, born from the Yoruba people of Nigeria, and origins anywhere between eight to ten thousand years old. My childhood home was deeply immersed in a diasporic branch of the Ifa and Orisa tradition, most commonly called Santeria. Ifa refers primarily to a canon of wisdom teachings, and Orisa refers to a variety of spiritual forces we might call deities. The Ifa tradition traveled to the Caribbean with the slave trade, and was syncretized with Catholicism so that the displaced people could continue their ancestral ways of worship. The term "Santeria" came from this syncretic element, as many of the ritualistic implements worked with at the time were hidden in catholic saints out of necessity. Another name for this diasporic expression, and less colored by this forced syncretic element, is La Regla De Ocha.

I was initiated into this tradition when I was a year and a half old. This is not common *at all*, as initiation into this tradition is quite demanding and formalistically extensive. While some details as to why I had to be initiated at such a young age are a little hazy, I am under the impression that through consulting various oracles, it was revealed that without initiation my life would end terribly early. My family initiated me to save my life. The word initiation is a bit overused nowadays, and in my opinion, many of its contemporary uses refer to relatively easy processes that do not amount to much. This is not the case in many of the old traditions, and is especially not true in La Regla De Ocha, as initiation requires tremendous engagement and sacrifice. There is much I cannot share for the sake of maintaining the integrity of these traditions, but I will share what I can to give a very small picture of a particular technology of consciousness, as expressed in one branch of one tradition. I will be very general and give highlights for the sake of simplicity. Henceforth, I will refer primarily to La Regla De Ocha; but please understand that the roots are *much* older, residing in the motherland of Africa and the Yoruba people.

To begin with, initiation into this tradition is not an event that we, as solo-practitioners, can just *choose to do* as independent agents. *Everything* in the tradition is mediated through a living, ongoing communication stream with powerful spirits. The otherworldly conversations take place through various forms of in-depth divination, carried out by elders. Actually, the regular use of oracles that are in communication with consistently responsive deities is a hallmark of the tradition. It puts the initiated person in a living stream of call and response processes.

To even be considered for initiation first requires connecting to spirits and investigating the appropriateness of doing so. A series of complex divinations are performed with one of the most extensive and intricate oracles on earth. These are not readings that one might get from any card reader out there. On their own, the divinations are vastly involved rituals with many prayers and calls to powerful, primordial forces. The traditional divinations set divinely attuned algorithms into motion that seek to understand the specifics of one's initiation. Great care is taken in knowing which deities' frequencies will be ritualistically activated within the individual. Once the divinations have given insight, clarity, and wisdom, the real work begins.

In general, the work requires between ten to twenty people to carry out, and the communal process can take multiple weeks to perform. Practical and spiritual preparation, as well as certain rituals for the individual about to undergo initiation starts a few days beforehand. The initiation itself is incredibly energy intensive, as it is a true mortal effort to touch both that which lies beyond and is also immanent. Multiple peak experiences occur during the communal effort to initiate the individual - and it's no wonder, as it is truly a process of being reborn.

Hundreds of plants are brought into the overall arc of the work - and this seems to be the case across many of the diasporic branches. A rich mix of diverse plants are utilized in very specific ways, and are prayed over with very particular prayers and songs in order to cleanse and consecrate various tools, shells, and containers/vessels. The level of plant knowledge the elders hold in the tradition is quite incredible! Initiations into La Regla De Ocha often require dozens of animal sacrifices, all of which are carefully carried out in a formulaic manner. This portion of the tradition may be difficult for outsiders to grasp; though, we have to understand that in Africa and in other places where branches of the tradition are practiced, this bloodshed is a natural extension of life and death. The blood, and at times other portions of the animal(s), are offered to the spirits, and the rest is eaten by the people in a sacred feast where humans and deities, together, eat the spoils of the hunt. There is no cruelty for cruelty's sake, and skillful, humane methods are the standard with these sacrifices. None of this is haphazard or lacking in nuance. It is not senseless or vulgar. *All* of it has a purpose.

The elders perform ritual bathing with the stews of plant medicines that have been prayed, chanted, and sung over. The initiate is cleansed, the head is shaved, and the body, from head to toe, is ceremoniously painted with a spectrum of colors. The songs, the blood, the plants, the chants, all of it, and all of the rituals come together in a deeply mesmerizing experience, and provide quite a spectacle for all of the senses. With everyone humming and singing along with the sacred songs, a sonic element is born and flows continuously throughout the protocol. People emotionally crack open from the powerful vibration that swirls around them. When the time comes, each of the deities are ushered into their own heavily consecrated porcelain or wooden pots. Each deity has their own protocols, rituals and mysteries for communion, and they each have their own shells, stones, or tools associated with them. Each deity receives their own oracle during initiation, as this helps to create a direct, reliable line of communication to them. For the active practitioner, this means of communication becomes a major hub of constant connection between them. To see this all happen is to witness gods being born.

After the intensive, multi-day process, with much of it being heated by such profound ritual activity, a cooling phase concludes the ceremony. The initiate resides in a dazzling, colorful throne-like structure made out of cloth for seven to ten days. Here, they rest, have quiet conversation, take time to reflect, and perhaps have periods of gentle celebration for what transpired. More rituals and life trajectory divinations are completed during this phase. From this moment on, the initiate only wears white clothing for one year, regardless of their job or life circumstances; and there's much more protocol that the initiate must follow once initiated. *This* is the doorway into the tradition; the beginning.

As expressed within one lineage of what is a powerful, and potentially, life-changing initiation, I have only scratched the surface. When the overall body of wisdom that is the Ifa and Orisa tradition is taken into account, initiation is a *tiny* piece of something that is incredibly vast and deep, that it boggles the mind. A lifetime could be spent studying this tradition and one would only learn a small fraction of what it contains. The degree of care, specificity, and formulaic considerations make it a very refined technology indeed. Although rituals often have practical considerations, rituals to create change in any number of worldly matters may also be included. Here, they seem to extend beyond that, as rituals in this tradition transform consciousness. It is challenging to go through an initiation as previously described without being changed. Whether that change can adhere to a person's core is another matter altogether. Yet, communion with the sacred, and the awakening of a more whole sense of being, is woven into technologies such as this.

In addition to undergoing this type of initiation as a small child, I too participated in ceremonies of initiation for dozens of others. I contributed by singing songs, preparing the plant medicines, cracking open coconuts, assisting with animal sacrifices, and butchering and preparing the carcasses as was required. My grandmother devoted her life exclusively to the tradition, and I by default, lived and breathed it with her. Divination, exorcisms, folk magic, and other ritual work is how she put food on our table. It is because of her that I had the privilege of learning how to do magic birthed from folk and Congolese methodologies.

I certainly am no authority in regards to the Ifa and Orisa tradition, and I have only shared *my own* exposure to a branch as I have understood it. However, I do believe that the Ifa and Orisa traditions are in fact one of the great spiritual wisdom traditions of the world, on par with anything found in the East or West. The *real* authorities of these traditions grow out of deep dedication, apprenticeship, and study. What I can say with certainty is that this tradition understands the primacy of consciousness and animism. They understand the living reality of primal forces, as they clearly take great strides in creating technologies to leverage and commune with them. While this specific tradition has its clear pathways and lineages about who can practice and perform what and when, this type of technology, although modified and changed in a number of ways within the diaspora, is an inheritance of an ancestral past from the Paleolithic era that was much more connected to the mystery. It's one expression of how the ancestors may have communed, practiced, and became ecstatic.

Something that is not readily apparent about this tradition, is that the tradition is actually monotheistic, and each of the deities is but one aspect, or emanation, of one god. The "many faces of god" as it were, expressing an immense totality that contains the spectrum of qualities. The one god, however, is considered a mystery beyond mortal human comprehension. In the same vein, divine destiny, the various mandates of heaven, and an ongoing connection to the god force within each of us, is also a core feature of the Ifa and Orisa tradition.

We are spiritual apes with parts of our brains and concurrent brain wave patterns devoted to divine, ecstatic connection. It is in our blood and in our bones. Fortunately for us, there are many paths to God through consciousness-based technologies available in many cultures. It is my assertion that connecting to divinity is a fundamental part of being human. By sharing a little about my own experience and lineage, I hope to illuminate this aspect of human heritage. We each have a sovereign right to engage with the divine in ways that speak to our unique essence. We each must find our own ways to pray and connect to potent practices meant to interweave our awareness with the divine. While, at times, organized religion-pathways may facilitate this connection, I encourage us to find ways to connect with the source of existence in tangible and embodied ways that flood our awareness and pours into our very being.

Magic Is Ancestral

In addition to our innate thirst for divine connection, we humans have a natural inclination to magic. There are so many traditions and magical paths that lead into the wilderness of the unseen, a domain difficult to domesticate. Yet, the majority of us have lost magic in our lives, as this is another limb that has been cut off from the human spirit. How are we to engage with something we were never taught to appreciate? It is truly up to each of us to find ways to satiate this hunger. We may be driven toward ancient, living traditions, or we may craft our own pathway. However we go about it, opening ourselves to re-engagement with a magical worldview may be profoundly nourishing for our spirits. Elements as simple as giving offerings to the dead; speaking to spirits of the land; donning magical charms, amulets, or talismans; and even praying over plants to create medicine can be considered magical. Nearly every culture on earth does this in some form or fashion. The human species is an animal with constant access to magic, as it appears to emerge from us regardless of the time or place we exist within.

Within the western culture, we are actively conditioned against the instinctual drive towards the mysterious and the miraculous. We even see this split in those who are interested in ancestral lifeways. In a general sense, they are interested in ancestral nutrition, circadian rhythms, natural light cycles, hunting and gathering, ancestral sexuality, and ancestral movement, yet they ignore the deep, magical aspects of the human lineage. The fragmentation happens in part because of the aforementioned conditioning, and in part due to science in the form of anthropology and archaeology. When examined under the severe and segregating gaze of a magnifying glass, the notion of magic having been practiced can be difficult. Science, in its current iteration, stands at the gates of the mind in staunch defense against what it considers "an archaic enemy to true knowledge." On the other side of that wall, contemporary magical circles tend to not be very illiterate in science, favoring the occult, and actively disregarding the value of the scientific process. Here, we have what can be classified as a war over how to perceive, and relate, to reality.

However, the disregard for the magical currents flowing underneath the "enlightened" and "rational" consensus the West swims in, stands in stark contrast to the ancestors who were decidedly immersed in a magical universe. In the broadest sense of the word, the ancestors were magicians. They engaged with practices and lifeworks which placed them in interaction with currents of unseen power, spirits, and magical forces. They knew a world full of gods and spirits, prayer, and places of power. The essence of nature breathed, pulsed, and at times, pounded within them with ferocious intensity. It is not uncommon to encounter living, indigenous medicine-people so profoundly immersed in the spirit world that blood literally pours from their noses. To them, these interactions are as real as gravity.

It is absolute hubris to hold the thousands of generations of humans who have come before us in contempt, as "superstitious savages that didn't know any better", and as "people decidedly lost and run amok in ignorance". Let us not pretend they lied in wait for the last, few dozen generations of humans to come and "correct their mistake." Although, it's surely not politically correct to state it - *that* is the unspoken weaving of thought under the surface of our culture. It's heartbreaking; for it brands our heritage and our innate nature as erroneous. It shoots the spirits of the ancestors at their core with an arrow of disregard. In turn, it makes us sick from our roots, up. Humans have performed rituals, danced wild and naked, and called upon the nectar of bliss, long before there was electricity. We crafted magical barriers to ward off phantasms that went bump in the night long before there was anti-virus software. We found potent allies in realms that could only be considered "other", long before social media.

Most of us have no real notion of where the source of this loss comes from, as it is unconscious. For if you do consider magic a superstitious impossibility, I ask if you even know where this disbelief originates from? Did it emerge out of your direct experience of the world or an unacknowledged binding you walked into? In all likelihood, it came from the culture you were brought up in, and conditioning; not an honest exploration of magical immersion. For most of us, this disbelief is a superficial set of ideas cultivated from the status quo, or words in a book, or characters in a movie.

In "The Chaos Protocols", magician, Gordon White, calls *having experiences that fundamentally shake your sacred, materialistic worldview view to its core,* as "becoming invincible"; or in his words: "Becoming invincible is the process of immunising yourself against the monoculture." Once we encounter certain forces, there is no going back. While Gordon has recommendations that go as far as advising someone (while simultaneously advising them against it) to spend a night in an abandoned mental hospital for accomplishing this immunization, the idea points towards something critical: the world we live in has been selectively sanitized of situations where we may encounter magic. Often, we must seek magic out and place ourselves in situations where we might directly meet the unbelievable, face-to-face.

CHAPTER 12

Reacquainting with Magical Culture

"Magic works in practice but not in theory"
- Peter J Carroll

"The Gods and spirits taught our ancestors and they can teach us as well." - John Beckett

Despite my obvious opinion that we humans are innately, a magical species, it is important for me to recognize that magical living can be a difficult prospect for many modern, western people. Not only does our culture push against its practice, there is deep trauma in the collective from the many practitioners of the past that were persecuted and devoured by the machinations of the church and its soldiers. The fear, the cries of anguish, the rage of loved ones being burned alive reverberates in time as an echo. Systems of power have also been put in place to prevent us from engaging with magic. Despite this, many of the most powerful individuals that come from old money, engage in occult rituals. No conspiracy theory here! Membership in certain occult orders is something that some of these families have openly admitted to. Even J.P. Morgan once famously said something to the effect of, "Millionaires don't need astrologers, but billionaires do." Far be it from these individuals to ignore the potential to exert more influence, regardless of its source.

The other matter is, that as a people, we do not have proper context for magical practices, whether in worldview or in technical application. Hollywood has certainly created unrealistic ideas that affect our perspective on what real magic is. Due to its influence on our perception of magic, we will miss the often subtle shifts in the webs of power and energy surrounding us if we only expect fireworks. This compounds our disbelief, but also adds expectations that simply cannot be met with consistency. Although it is possible, rarely does magic involve lightning shooting down from the sky. More often than not, magic occurs in the quiet spaces of a personal altar, or in simple communion with natural forces.

If we hold onto notions of what magic is supposed to be like, we miss what it actually is due to not being present with the in-the-moment reality. Even still, when approaching the living veins of magical traditions still being practiced today, we may feel stifled just by knocking on the front door. The Ifa and Orisa tradition is an excellent example of this, as the tradition has been passed down from generation to generation for thousands of years. All of its branches are heavily protocol-based, and in some ways, can be incredibly rigid in implementation. I don't assume I know all of the reasons for this, but among the viable reasons, it is to make the tradition highly transmissible to others with minimal loss of effectiveness.

If it were a free-for-all, it wouldn't have survived across millennia. Safety and a strong reliance on repeatability have been created through the time-tested protocols; and it should be so considering that they are dealing with intensely powerful spirits! There are huge consequences when practicing magic at such high levels. In addition to established procedures, the tradition has hierarchies in place; secrets are dished out as one ascends in the hierarchy; and only until deemed ready by elders, one is taught highly technical skills. While all of this preserves potency, and effectiveness, it can limit approachability, especially in a modern context. Of course, this is just one example, as many established traditions have apparent ways of working with magic, and a wide variety of qualifiers for even being allowed to do so.

Then we have the proverbial "witch in the woods" traditions: those that may speak to a somewhat, more wild, free, and explorative relationship to magic. This shadowy domain belongs to the solo-practitioner, or to small secret groups that often learn directly from spirits. This approach requires a great dose of trial-and-error, and often involves getting one's fingers burned. Practitioners in these circles can develop highly nuanced and idiosyncratic ways of working magic that produce immense power and effectiveness. Often, these systems are not highly transmissible, though they may be passed down to some degree within certain families or circles. These systems often die with the death of those who practice them, or in other cases, simply do not work well for others.

There are those who merge both paths. Those individuals are generally thoroughly trained, and are exceptionally capable magicians, who often end up diving head-first into magic, happily swimming in multiple currents with gusto. My grandmother was such a person. While she was a highly trained initiate in La Regla De Ocha, she also had a very alive, smokey, rich, and powerful, spirit-based practice that heavily relied on direct transmission with the spirits. She relied on her exceptionally capable practice to do work for others and for her own needs. This particular path requires a willingness to engage, and to a degree, trust in that that is not common.

Regardless of the chosen path, and despite some results with magic that do not require much skill, it must be understood that reliable and powerful magic is a skillset. Effective magicians attempt to get better with time, and to be an effective magician requires dedication, study, and much experimentation. For those who start out, the first real challenge will be in finding the real thing as they may encounter many charlatans and mediocre practitioners.

To add to the difficulty of engaging with magic in modern times, we must also consider the inner state of the person seeking magic in their life. Beliefs, personal issues, emotional wounds, trauma, and conditioned patterns may not align with the fundamental nature of magic. Few understand that to be a magician, will often require serious internal work, and, like the Phoenix, die again and again, in the fire of the magical path. If rebirth does not occur, then magic cannot be expected to work well over the long term.

Although there is much to recommend it, the reawakening of magical culture does not, by necessity, require one to be a deeply skilled magical practitioner interested in developing higher degrees of power. It is not dependent on one joining a magical tradition either. There will always be those who take things further, in their dedication, in their goals, and so on. What the majority of us may find we love though, is to let magic breathe back into daily life, and to acknowledge the existence of forces beyond the material; to remember that spirits lurk in the bushes of our yards, or that plant people respond to simple prayers. We can acknowledge the mystery of existence while actively engaging with it.

All of this can be as simple as tending to an ancestral shrine, or giving an offering to spirits once a week. At some level, magic is a part of all of us by simply being human. We need not be intimidated by our lack of magical context, nor by what is required to have serious magical skill. Simple and direct ways to begin living alongside the magical currents once again, and awakening a sense of awe and wonder is what may lead to more wholeness right now. Many cultures still live in this way. Even though our culture actively suppresses that in us, we can begin to wake up, and create a culture where magic is real and a part of how we live. In so doing, we would be deeply honoring our ancestors and our nature. I wholeheartedly recommend anyone who is interested in approaching magic to read Aidan Wachter's book, "Six Ways."

Practices for Relating to the Internal and External

"The great majority of men in cities are apt to pride themselves on their own exemption from 'superstition' and to smile pityingly at the poor countrymen and countrywomen who believe in fairies. But when they do so they forget that, with all their own admirable progress in material invention, with all the far-reaching data of their acquired science, with all the vast extent of their commercial and economic conquests, they themselves have ceased to be natural." - Walter Yeeling Evans-Wentz

Although, currently, my recommendation to those interested in beginning a magical practice is to check out "Six Ways", I did want to offer an elementary way for readers to begin engaging with the world from an animist perspective in relation to magic. Beginning to cultivate a type of sensory experience may feed into magic, or it may simply enrich your sense of the world around you. It is incredibly helpful to step out of the excessive reliance on rational and intellectual methods of knowing. This is not to say that our intellect is a lesser aspect of being; it's just that these faculties are a primary barrier in our culture, and often have to undergo a rebirthing process to be helpful magical allies. Here, it is best to immerse oneself in direct experience of consciousness and human flesh living in relationship with the world around us.

The following exercises goes beyond what many people may label as intuition and is simply a type of perception. To be honest, intuition is a nuanced skill set that is not very developed in most modern people. There is deep discernment needed to make intuition work at a functional level, and it's certainly not a practice that is cultivated in most. With that being said, the following will be a way to take in information and act on it; to perceive the underlying, qualitative flows of organic energy and consciousness present with what is mistakenly referred to as inanimate.

The modern mind tends to run into the desire for scientific certainty; however, this type of work is purely relational. If personhood can be extended to plants, minerals, animals, ideas, myths, gods, and even man-made objects, such as cars, computers, and houses, then the type of information we receive is relative to our particular relationship with said person. Any and all of the various dynamics about how humans engage with one another can be applied to animist-relational dynamics. The interpersonal dynamics, conversations, and emotional dances of relating can never be expressed with scientific exactness, or in many ways, even considered objective.

Feelings and attitudes that emerge in shared connections will flow, shift, change, grow, ruminate, explode, and subside in an ongoing tango that includes the stories of all sides. For example, your spouse may show up differently for you than they would for their boss, yet they're being authentic in expressing who they are. Someone may behave differently toward those within their own ethnic groups due to the degree of understanding that underlies that particular group, and yet, won't, and can't, replicate that behavior within other ethnic groups. A relationship of five years that has seen and overcome immense struggle, might be more profound than one of 15 years that has been more superficial in nature. All of this is the same in animist relationships. Once we understand that, it will be easy to see why a person's relationship to a particular herb, stone, deity, or land spirit may be very different from ours.

To experience the world as an animist is to immerse oneself in an ongoing dialogue that is dynamic, adaptable, and responsive; to be with all of it; and to know that to perceive is to be *in* relationship, in and of itself. To do this, we need to rely on something deeper and wiser than intellectual standards. Here is where we begin to sense through our bellies and our bones, and relate to them as primal antennae that pick up on the underlying currents of energy. The belly has no eyes, but it can feel its way through the world through vibration, temperature, texture, and quality, just like an earthworm can. The bones are much like tuning forks, capable of resonating and vibrating in their own way. These are ancient, perceptive faculties that can offer us a type of information that can be very useful to us. We can begin to work with these faculties to explore a wider net of relationships, and even begin building particular relationships if we choose. We will want to open up our perceptual capacities beyond the mind, and will do well to not become overly mechanical with this practice.

Listening with the Belly and Bones:

1. Find a place where you can be undisturbed and feel at ease. This can be in nature or in your home.
2. Take a herb, stone, small plant, or some other natural object (it is much easier to start with natural objects at first) and bring the item to your navel area.*
3. As in the "Activating Primal Consciousness" exercise, swallow your awareness into your belly. From here, feel into the space between your belly and the person you are holding.
   - What impressions do you get?
   - Do you see any colors?
   - What emotions, temperature, quality, texture, ideas, or inspirations move through you?
4. Now, fill in the gap, and sense the person you're holding directly. Follow the same process, taking in all of the information you receive. Treat it like a conversation.
5. As you get more comfortable, attempt to sense with your bones. The bones in the thighs and arms are often easier to sense with for most. Eventually, you'll want to bring your whole skeletal structure into the sensing.
6. From this place of sensing with the bones and with the belly, connected as one sense organ, what do you receive?

*A note: please be aware of the qualities of the stone or plant you choose, such as knowing whether or not you're allergic to them, or whether they're poisonous or potentially toxic. It would be wise to verify this before you consider touching them with your body in any capacity. This type of perception does not replace common sense and the realities of the world.

Direct Relating:

Along the same lines as the previous exercise, this is a basic approach to internal awareness to begin to relate to what is happening within as *alive*. Emotions, thoughts, sensations, and other qualities may have a type of life or personality that we can engage with directly. It is important to acknowledge that many in our modern world are numb to the internal sensations, and the overall quality of experiences moving through them. Even still, having a way to relate beyond mere reaction or unconsciousness to the inner universe is critical.

If we can perceive something, we may be able to change it; it is difficult to shift and engage with something if we can perceive it. This exercise is a way of developing a better sense of relating capacity with our internal sensations and experiences, and helps us take on an animist stance on the world within. It will especially be helpful if we run into uncomfortable sensations moving within us, although, it can definitely be applied to neutral and pleasurable feelings as well.

Overtime, feel free to refine the following sequence to your own needs:

1. Go to a place where you can sit or lay down quietly, and be undisturbed.
2. Feel into your body and find the sensation you want to engage with.

3. Immediately create an impression of space around the sensation. Although it may take some time, let go of any tightening or constriction that may pop up.
4. Begin to soften around the sensation. Soften your mind and soften your spirit. A helpful awareness to play with here may be that of melting the tension around the sensation.
5. Begin to perceive and describe the feeling(s) in a qualitative manner.
   - What is its color, overall texture, temperature, and size? *This can be anything, such as volcanic, electric; deep, crimson in color; a size that goes far beyond the body. It could also be tiny, gray, and feel numb, or it could feel cold and spinning in place.*
   - Does it have any movement patterns?
6. Now, if you can, begin to question the sensation and simply listen.
   - Ask how it is trying to help you.
   - What does it want? Why is it there?
7. Then try to negotiate with it, or, if needed, ask it to shift in a certain way. Engage in dialogue with the sensation the way you would with a person.

CHAPTER 13

Necromancy to Better the Living

"These practices may be disturbing to some and it is wise to remember: we are all here due to the dead that came before us. The very nutrients in the soil we grow our food in are created by the process of death and decay. Even to clear a field to grow grains or beans on, destroys a vast number of lifeforms inhospitable to the process of farming. There is no life without dying. There is no birth without death."
- Aidan Wachter in "Six Ways"

"So long as you do not die and rise again, you are a stranger to the dark earth." - Goethe

In some ways, this book carries necromantic undertones to it. Unfortunately, that word carries negative connotations. We can probably thank Hollywood a bit for skewing our perception of something that is so natural for us, and for degrading anything that is occult by associating them with things of evil and demonic workings. Of course, there are significant occult fields of study around the subject that may include some serious and terrifying work. By definition, though, necromancy simply means working with the dead, and in a lot of ways, this book asks us to actively engage with the dead in order to have a clearer connection to life. When we look at the past, engage with those who have died in order to learn, grow, and become more whole, we are practicing necromancy. In fact, when done properly, certain types of necromantic work can help life to flourish. Although the word may carry fear and mystique, for many, elements of it are absolutely accepted in our present day. One of the basic and cross-culturally accepted forms of necromancy would be the purposeful burying of the dead. Should it be a surprise that this is something our ancestors did as well? Some of the oldest burial rites that have been found, by current estimates, occurred anywhere between 70 to 80 thousand years ago; and they likely took place for much longer than that.

Whether we acknowledge it or not, the dead are all around us. The dead are in the food we eat, they are in the land we build our house on, they are in the systems left behind by previous generations, they are in the language we speak today, they are in the inherited patterns of our lineage; and they are the fossil fuels that power our technology. The dead pervasively impact us.

Yet, death has been sanitized from our world. We no longer have a visceral experience of death. For the most part, death now takes place in hospital rooms and nursing homes. Many of us are no longer involved in the killing of an animal for food and resources; and those who have to, and *will* kill an animal out of mercy, are few and far between. Many ancestors watched the last breath be drawn by beings that were going to be eaten or by loved ones whose time had come. Death was intimate. A breath of gratitude over the fresh kill or a gathering of the tribe as an elder prepared to step out of their human body, allowing all the opportunity to say their blessings and educating the young on what was occurring without filter.

Today, with our rigid, cold walls and fluorescent lights, we lack a solid relationship with death; we have become strangers to it. In this, we've lost the edge that gives life its sharpness, as knowing death sharpens the sense of life; it offers lucidity and crispness to what life is. It may come off as an odd thing to state: but I think most people would do well to be involved with the humane killing of an animal to feed themselves; or to be involved in a mercy kill of an animal who is irreparably injured rather than letting it suffer; or to be involved in the compassionate euthanasia of a senior animal in need of assistance. If not involving oneself with these real and necessary forms of death, perhaps they would do well to volunteer in the spaces that see death continually, such as nursing homes, hospice centers, and funeral parlors. Relating-to-death practices such as these are extreme, sure, but they are not uncommon in many parts of the world. Some direct experience with death, even if just minor, is a necessary part of developing a more complete view of the living.

In addition to no *real* relationship with death, we have learned to make an enemy of death, largely due to fear. We fear dissolution, the loss of control it denotes, the stark loneliness of dying, and for many, the terror of the dark unknown. I cannot say I have no fear of death, but I can say that it is a conscious practice to make peace with it while doing my best not to hide from death. One thing that helps me is knowing that the fear of death is actually the fear of life - for until we can trust in death, we cannot fully trust in life. Carl Jung said, "Not wanting to live is synonymous with not wanting to die. Becoming and passing away are the same curve." and "Whoever does not accompany the curve remains suspended in the air and grows numb."

The death card in some tarot decks has also helped me look at death in a different light. "Death" is spinning its scythe in an eternal dance of change and transformation. It is this essence of change that is required to remain in-touch with life. Without change, we become frozen and stuck within patterns that have lost their aliveness. We become less responsive to the new versions of ourselves trying to emerge, and we shut them down for a fear of losing something we have identified with for long periods of time. Change and transformation requires death to happen. If we learned to slowly make a friend of death, it would allow for more life to flow into our world; and when the time to face death comes, we'd know that we truly lived. In reference to the death card, Sallie Nichols wrote the following in the book, "Jung and Tarot":

> *"It represents the bare bones of reality; the scaffolding for our flesh and muscles, the jointed framework upon which everything else hangs together, moves and functions as a whole unit. And yet, paradoxically, this instrument of change also represents our most enduring part. It is the body self that we leave behind for future historians – the sole testimony of existence as individuals. It is all that remains of our ancestors – of our roots buried deep in time. The skeleton is the archetypal Homo sapiens."*

Is it any surprise that death and the ancestors often conjure up visions of a skeleton, and that many ancestral shrines are decorated with bones and skulls? With all of that being said, to work with the dead healthfully, we *will* be asked to examine the relationship we have to death and dying. Again, we don't need to disregard life in accepting death in this way; quite the opposite. We can cultivate a vibrant relationship to life *and* death, and understand that they are two poles of the same spectrum. In fact, many who have had near death experiences are permanently shaken and return, not with dread, but with a stronger appreciation for being alive and are more at peace. For them, to have peered through death's door, and to have seen the radiant world beyond the flesh, was profoundly healing. *This* realm, beyond the flesh, is the resting place of the ancestors.

Ancestral Tending

"Death is an intelligent and organized process."
- Dr. James Jealous, D.O.

Now we will explore what is likely to be one of the oldest forms of devotional practice in our human story: the veneration and healthful tending of the dead. In one form or another, we as a species have engaged with reverence of our ancestors and the "mighty dead" for millennia. (The "mighty dead" show up as patrons of living traditions; as saints, avatars, royalty, and in some cases, deities.) Ancestral veneration is a time-honored and cross-cultural practice around the globe. It can take on many forms, but at its basic level, ancestral veneration is the acknowledgment of the dead that have come before us as ever-present, *and* that those who come after us will have to contend with what *we* have left behind. The ancestral cycle moves from cradle to grave. We, ourselves, are a part of this cycle and in turn, become ancestors. We could not be here without them, just as future generations cannot be without us. We all belong to one another and are bound through time. We are a part of a continuum moving forward and backward through time, anchored in the here and now.

As individuals, and as a society, we can encounter many issues by not having practices for easing and appeasing the dead. Some of our ancestors may try to "live through us" in ways that are not helpful, and other problems can arise when the dead are not properly tended to. Few things are as meaningful to us as the bonds we build with our loved ones. If we can extend this sense of bond beyond the visibly alive and into the direct experience of ancestral engagement, we can heal massive rifts caused by the loss of this tradition. From my own experience, I have found the ancestors to be very present. Rebuilding a connection to them was not always easy, but it has been rewarding, clarifying, and deeply nourishing.

Typically, there is a need for most westerners to harmonize content that possesses an ancestral origin. I can say, from experience, that it will be helpful to begin addressing the spiritual currents flowing through our lives as we begin to solidify the ancestral connections in our lived experience through the practices outlined so far. Ancestral tending is a core practice to be recommended to *anyone* interested in ancestral lifeways. Many of our wounds, habits, impulses, and perceptions are not just our own; they are patterns that have been inherited through our lineage at one time or another. Yes, we can absolutely shift these patterns without having to address the ancestors, but recurring issues that do not seem to budge, often have a transpersonal element to them. However, it must be stated, that what is presented herein, cannot address the larger topics of ancestral healing, ancestral karma, working magic with the ancestors, and harmonizing the different lines together. In order for us to keep our expectations in alignment with the goal of *this* section, let us remember that this is about *beginning* our approach. The following will also give us direct access (albeit at a basic level) to addressing unhealthy patterns inherited from our ancestral line that may flow into conscious awareness.

A Deep Wellspring of Support, and Bindings and Curses

"The ghosts are baked into the system..."
- Daniel Foor

We must accept that in the world of relationships, we embrace that which is helpful and that which is unhelpful in varying quantities. Often, we are not given something that is pristine and endlessly helpful, without needing to rumble with some challenging elements in turn. Life carries a price of resistance. Challenge and support flow and weave together as one. This is the case in both relationships with the living and with the dead. When we take the time to dig the well, the ancestors can be a deep wellspring of support. At its health-oriented core, the ancestral domain can be extremely supportive, loving, and nourishing. Our success is their success. The ancestors are deeply invested in us, for we are the tip of the spear of our ancestral line. It is through our ongoing thriving that we can fulfill the desire and drive of our line. If we can orientate the ancestral line toward the auspicious, it can be immeasurably beneficial in our lived experience.

In regards to ancestral tending, Gordon White has said, "this is the best luck magic there is", and I have to agree with that, as my life has changed for the better, in numerous practical ways, since starting my own ancestral veneration practice! However, to unlock this quality of improving our lives through ancestral tending, we must heal the line.

Both love and pain echo through generations. Bindings and cursings exist within our ancestral lines that we have to dissolve or exorcize in order to shift the ratio of their impact on health and vibrancy. Curses can include unresolved drives or desires; traumas; genetic illnesses; troubled, hungry ghosts who are evolutionary mismatches with modern life; and inherited familial patterns. Although real, literal familial curses are not as common. Many unresolved or persistent negative patterns effectively behave like curses or bindings.

We heal the line, not just for our own wellbeing, but for the line itself. It is not unheard of for dynamics to begin to shift within a family in response to this healing work. I've noticed it upon numerous occasions within my own healing work. Support is readily available to us within the line because it already has radiant, bright ancestors at the ready to begin the reconciliation process; some of it has to be worked for by clearing up some static first. Fortunately, we already have access to a few ways to begin to do this, such as engaging in primal movements; activating our primal consciousness; through ancestral nutrition; and other aspects of ancestral life we've touched on already.

Curses and binding often travel through families over many generations, insidiously finding perches within our heritage. Let's call it "bad blood"; this "bad blood" of energetic and behavioral patterns does not arrest just us, as individuals; they bind us all to each other through time. Our ancestors dealt with their own version of the curses/bindings, and now we're dealing with it. Whether we are even aware of it or not, some wounding, habits, or perceptions experienced by our great- great- great-grandparents (and/or beyond), slowly traveled through the generations and have made its way to us, expressing itself in our modern world. At times, the curses/bindings can be beliefs or attitudes that have been conditioned into us at an early age. At other times, they may emerge from an ancestral ghost or a genetic memory. For example, for women I know, the women in their families experienced sexual trauma over generations; this in turn influenced how they related to their own sexuality, and that then impacted what they taught their own daughters about sex. These influences affect their own sexuality, their relationships to men, and their overall sense of desire. This is just one example, but the principle can extend to almost any element of human life.

A personal example of a binding/curse in my own line relates to currency and resources. My great-grandfather on my maternal side was one of the wealthiest men in Cuba before the infamous, Fidel Castro, arrived and through military force, took over the island. My family lost everything they had worked for in this ordeal. My family went from having mansions with in-house staff and owning multiple businesses, to fleeing the country and arriving in Miami with nothing to their name. My great-grandfather died in the U.S. from cancer, in a state of poverty. Without question, all of this has impacted my own relationship with money. It mostly shows up through a fear of having more of it, around losing it, and the pain that would come from such a fall.

Beyond the impact on my emotional and mental relationship with money, I've noticed its more "magical" effects on me. An example where this became blatantly obvious to me was when I underwent the process of opening my first brokerage account. This process, which usually takes no longer than 20 minutes, turned into a massive time-consuming ordeal. I was standing in the lobby of the bank with two bank tellers, completely at a loss about what was occurring, unsure of what to do next. They showed me their computer screen to see if I could figure it out, and that's when I felt my great-grandfather's spirit - and his fear. His voice roused up inside of me, warning me of potential losses and the pain of losing so much. It was utterly unbelievable. In seconds, I could feel the wounds that form from working your whole life to build your life, only to have it all taken from you in a blink of an eye, by no fault of your own. I went outside, and I spoke with him earnestly from the heart. It wasn't until then that the issue resolved itself. I went back into the bank, and just a few minutes later, I had my first brokerage account. The missing link ended up being a type of bank account connection needed to allow money to be freely transferred between two accounts. A situation that went from, "We have no idea what is going on here." to, "Aha! This should work."

Ancestral curses and bindings can affect us beyond the internal or behavioral levels. At times, they can extend beyond the self and into the material world. Why or how this happens, isn't important here. What is important, is the recognition that we *may* have the responsibility of dancing with these types of inheritances. If we are able to tend to them honestly, perhaps over a period of time, beautiful gifts can begin to emerge.

Maintaining Sovereignty and Avoiding The Traps of Time

If we are engaged in the work of connecting to ancestral forces, and developing an ancestral veneration practice, knowing how to maintain sovereignty is a critical skill. By virtue of being dead, does not turn one into an all-knowing-being or saint. We must interact with spiritual forces the way we would with a human being: by cultivating relationships that have a two-way feedback loop and that honors the freedom of each individual. We are not required to do what they tell us to; though we absolutely can, if that is what we choose to do.

I've noticed that handing over our sovereignty to spiritual forces is a common theme in some circles. Unless one enjoys being haplessly bounced around by disembodied beings, it is likely a major mistake to do so. It would be wise to remember that we are also spiritual beings - beings of consciousness that live here and now, perfectly capable of being responsible for our own lives. However, by entering into a relationship with spirits, by default, we are bringing them into our lives and entering into a two-way communication system. The spirits get to have their input; and they have their own preferences and may have their own idiosyncrasies. Just like with people in our world, the degree of how spirits impact and affect our world is a matter of defining the relationships and our boundaries.

Another consideration to take around ancestral veneration would be engaging in unhealthy forms of cultural conservatism. There are reasons to maintain cultural heritage alive, but let's not pretend that this is universal. An extreme but useful example would be Nazis: cultural lines can carry prejudice, racism, hate, anger, and other toxic bedfellows. There are aspects of cultures that arose out of necessity back in time, yet are not circumstances that are helpful to us today. While we may be ready to shed some of these practices, some of our ancestors may not be. We have no obligation to take these qualities on for ourselves, nor do we need to feed them into our ancestral veneration practices. Simply put, it is wise not to feed into their own undoing.

Personally, this is a main reason why I orientate my practice toward the whole of ancestry, rather than just recent ancestry. I do not leave out my recent ancestry, but I do not overly engage in that area outside of ancestral lineage healing. Everyone interested in ancestral veneration will have their own practice, and everyone will have to make their own judgment calls and take responsibility for how they venerate.

When we begin to engage with ancestral forces and the structures they built, a risk that we may run into is getting stuck, becoming frozen in time. This can happen in a number of ways, and in each case, our aliveness erodes. One example is tradition: by continuing to do something that may no longer serve our work or our lives, purely because "it has always been done this way." Granted, there are traditions that have stayed alive, need not be changed, and continue to serve the purpose they were created for, while continuously transferring its hard-won wisdom through the ages. These traditions are akin to the shark, in which evolutionary forces have repetitively weighed over eons of time, and have found them to be up to par as they are.

It's the traditions that masquerade as vital and alive but suppress forward movement that we must be wary of. They are energy-intensive shrines to old ideas whose time has come and passed. Just because something is old does not make it useful. Some traditions need to be allowed to pass away with grace, because propping them up is like being a puppeteer for a corpse.

A good way to know if we are in a tradition that no longer has vibrancy or use, is by examining the amount of work required for the degree of results that is achieved by the majority of its practitioners, and whether that makes sense to us to continue engaging in at a deeper level.

Another way is by knowing what one is seeking, as this is part of understanding the value of a tradition. For instance, there are many old martial arts that require five to ten years of consistent, daily practice before certain movements can be applied in real life; while more contemporary expressions of the combative arts may be applied in 6 months. There are many reasons to practice old martial arts, and there are many that are not combat related. If one was to consider taking up a martial arts practice, it would do them well to consider all of these expressions and weigh what would be most beneficial to them, and if that particular tradition would feed into the aliveness they want to feel. Without question, natural forces appreciate efficiency, and do not seem to be wasteful of energy when at all possible.

Another way we can become frozen in time is by accepting the status quo. If we do so, we end up leading unexamined lives, akin to wearing outfits that someone else laid out for us before we awoke. Mushtaq Al Ali Ansari has often said, "Disobedience is an act of spiritual hygiene." It took me a long time to understand that this quote went beyond disobeying momentary circumstances and extended through time. We must be willing to accept the value offered to us by the past, while also judiciously dissolving that which no longer offers value, without apology. I find this to be a useful way to honor our ancestors.

We must learn to relate to ancestral forces in a manner that is not limiting but empowering. Consider that traditions were created in an attempt to solve a problem, or to pass on storehouses of knowledge and wisdom that could generate solutions. If they no longer do that, we must become like our ancestors, shed old skin, and do the same for our future generations. By and large, the ancestors have been innovators; this can be seen from the discovery of fire to its more modern rendition found in the sparks of technology. The consistent drive to discover, create, invent, and improve is a part of human inheritance. Turning the established order on its head and applying the heat of transformation is a defining key feature of who we are. This is what I mean when I say we must become like our ancestors in regards to tradition - recognizing that structures are built, and they are subsequently torn down, or parts are recreated, and that it is all part of a natural cycle of change and stability bouncing off of each other. Many of us seem rather attached to the stability side of the cycle; likely due to the energy-conserving properties of keeping things the same, since growth often ruffles the feathers of ingrained patterns, and requires high outputs of energy initially. So while we tune into the much older and innate aspects of our being, let's also be conscious of the fact that the act of improvement is also innate.

Before we move on, here are a few questions to mull over:

Identify three to five traditions that you inherited from your family or culture. Can you tease out what their purpose may have been when they were created? Are the traditions still accomplishing their purpose now? Lastly, what traditions are we collectively holding onto that need to be let go?

CHAPTER 14

Starting an Ancestral Veneration Practice

"It seems like getting back to the source of life, whether that's Eden or Asgaard - is about a return to family. Not sole fame. It's all about the weight of our relationships. And if bliss in our afterlife is seeing those we loved or joining the other ones we fought with - then most of our tales are of a spiritual reunification with a community, a people."
- Eric Haggstrom

To begin with, unless one has access to clear instructions from a trustworthy source, I would not suggest building a shrine for the ancestors. Any shrine or altar anchors something's power into the physical world more fully and creates a node for that force. Due to this, the shrine becomes a living being and requires commitment and maintenance. While useful, shrines are not necessary for connecting with ancestral forces. Honestly, it could be argued that the lineage carried within our bodies is the strongest living shrine of our ancestors.

Starting a relationship with the ancestors does not need to be incredibly complex, but it does require some knowledge and a few skills that many of us in the modern world do not possess. Encountering forces within the ancestral currents that are wounded, traumatized, or sick in some way pose a real danger. Although these forces do exist, so do the healthy ancestral forces that can be protective agents for us if we engage with them intelligently. We have to remember that we are the tip of the spear when it comes to our ancestors. Our entire heritage that came before us, lies within us. The ancestors have a vested interest in our being prosperous, because as we prosper, so does the whole lineage. So, although there is that danger, excessive fear is not really warranted in most situations.

How To Call The Ancestors

My advice for calling in the ancestors, especially at first, is to have some qualifiers. We don't want to call on "everyone who is willing to show up." Just as one would be discerning as to who to invite to their house or wedding, one would do well to be smart with who they're calling in from the ancestral line, and what type of ancestors one is calling in. We do this with the language we use in our calls. Regardless of whatever deeper mystery the ancestor spirits actually are, the way *we* orient toward them will make a large difference in the type of experiences we will have.

Here are some examples of useful language to work with:
I call upon ancestors who bring wisdom, beauty, truth, love, support, vibrancy, and guidance.

...ancestors who accept me and appreciate me.

...ancestors who are full of light and radiance.

...ancestors who are healthy and well in spirit.

...ancestors who bring protection, warmth, and clarity.

Here is a sample prayer to draw inspiration from:
From this nexus point in time, from this place here and now, I call upon the ancestors who bring love, beauty, and truth. I call upon the ancestors who bring light, love, and radiance. I call upon the ancestors who bring support, wisdom, and guidance. Stretching back and forward through time, a call goes out to those of you who accept and love me. May we sit together, commune, and share this space.

The theme of the examples is calling upon spirits who will, for the most part, be harmonious, healing, and supportive to us. We want to call upon spirits that are primarily well. This language will provide a simple, yet safe and straight-forward means of engagement.

It may be helpful to know that one can feel the presence of healthy ancestral forces. Before I was ever officially taught it, it was always my experience that healthy, vibrant ancestors often showed up as beings of radiant light. I later found that this was a common experience for others, and is even in teachings from well-known teachers of this work. Others may experience an immediate response as a sudden overwhelm of emotion, which is a common effect of legitimate spirit contact. Others may not feel anything immediate. Some may feel fireworks the first time they do this and others may call several times before feeling it. A large part of feeling the response depends on how cultivated one is in sensing subtle phenomena, one's personal disposition, dominant senses, and so on.

A properly crafted ancestral practice is one of the least risky, and most beneficial means of consorting with spirits, but it must be mentioned that consorting with spirits always carries a risk. Nothing in life is 100% safe; there are always dangers. Welcome to being alive! However, in the case of engaging with the ancestors, the rewards outweigh the risk. Be smart. The odds are strongly in your favor. Unless one runs into serious trouble, in which case, seeking out help from someone qualified is wise, I would stay consistent with this practice.

For the sake of specificity in ancestral veneration, it is useful to define the classes of ancestors. The ancestral spectrum is as follows:

The Human Ancestors - *remembered dead, deep lineage, collective dead*:

This class includes what most people think of when they think of ancestors. These are the remembered dead - the people of our most recent ancestry. This is the tip of the gargantuan iceberg that leads us through biblical times, through the beginning of civilization, and all the way back to the first human beings. This is the domain of Homo sapiens proper. It is a critically important element of our ancestry and is very diverse. A rainbow of different times, places, traditions, cultures, and people somehow all originating from a few conception points. Of course, with all of that diversity, this sphere of ancestors can clearly have helpful beings, and those that are unhelpful. This is why it is important to have a clear way to partition vital spirits from the wounded, especially when first starting out with ancestral veneration.

Deep Ancestors - *pre-human, mythological, the animals:*

The Deep Ancestors include all the non-human ancestry going back to the first lifeforms in the primeval oceans. This is an enormous family tree that includes worms, fish, reptiles, early mammals, primates, and proto-humans or other hominids. This sphere has mythological components related to deep, primal forces in nature - this is where ideas about particular clans being related to elements or animals come into play. From a more contemporary perspective, it could be said that certain lineages relate to various archetypal or genetic forces. A slightly more esoteric view point would see the intermingling of entities and lineage ancestors at some point in the deep past. Whatever the truth is, there are strong wild forces in the deep ancestry. From a proper vantage point, the stars could also be considered ancestors, for we are literally made of stardust. Our solar system star, the sun, makes life possible and the light it shines on this planet flows through each of us.

Although these ancestors can be called upon, I would first establish a strong and healthy practice with the human ancestors first. When one is feeling safe and ready to do so, here is a language sample that you can rework to your liking to call upon the Deep Ancestors:

> *I call out to the ancestors stretching back to the ancient oceans, all the way back to the first life forms on this planet. I call out to the animals of my lineage and heritage. The creatures of the earth that led into and became humanity. I call out to the primal and primordial forces of my ancestral line. I call out to the stars and the mythological forces within my line.*

Spiritual Ancestors - *spiritual lineage, the deeply loved dead:*
The Spiritual Ancestors are related to those beings who have deeply impacted our world through our spirit or consciousness. This may be through spiritual traditions that one happens to be a part of, through deep resonance with people from the past - and can even be those one has never met, or those who were our chosen family members who are now dead. This sphere is not invested in the genetic lineage. For example, my wife holds that an Arctic wolf, named Storm, whom she cultivated a close relationship with for about five or more years at the

wolf sanctuary, is a spiritual ancestor of hers. She has multiple wolves or wolfdogs in this sphere of ancestors. However, one does not need to be very specific here. I am usually not, yet I do honor this lineage knowing that whoever needs to hear it, will.

Giving Offerings

Once a connection with the ancestors has been made, and by either having made the call or having received a response, giving offerings and communing with them is the next stage. Giving spirits offerings in some form is pretty much standard practice the world over. It is most commonly seen in indigenous cultures, but many other cultures who are connected to the modern world still do so. Offerings provide the spirits with food, nourishment, and strengthening, as well as helping to grease the grooves, so to speak, of the interaction. It also aids in building the relationship while providing them a touchstone in the physical world that thereby provides them energy.

Offerings can do many things, and can even be worked with as a whole system of magic in itself. In this case, though, we will keep it simple. My suggestion is to offer candles, water, and incense as a basic starting place. After the ancestors are called, I let them know that I am giving them offerings to nourish them, strengthen them, and appease them. By doing so, I am acknowledging that they are remembered, honored, and appreciated - and that is healing for them. If offering a candle, always practice safety. When the candle has finished burning (generally a good idea to use a tealight), or when you have to put out the flame, it is a good idea to let them know that you are removing the offering. In the case of water, it is unwise to let the water sit for days, or allow it to turn. It is a polite thing to let them know that you are removing the offering.

Communion

Communion with the ancestors can be very simple. Simply begin by speaking to them from the heart. You can share your day with them, what's currently on your mind; your worries, concerns, desires, joys, and treasures; you can express gratitude for the gift of life. Communing with them can be as simple as connecting to a close, loved, and trusted friend. Once you have shared, sit quietly and listen. Just be present. Be open to the physical sensations, sights, sounds, smells, and tastes that crop up in the silence. Some may experience all types of sensorial aspects, and others may not feel much - either case is fine. Just setting the intention to listen is enough. Something I enjoy doing from time to time is to make a cup of tea with a little extra and go sit with the ancestors. I offer them a shot glass of the tea and sip on my own tea without making a big deal out of it. I may call upon them in a relaxed and easy-going manner. Mostly, I just calmly speak to them and share in the joy of a cup of tea.

Once a relationship has been established and you feel supported by them, you can call on them in times of difficulty and pain. There is a deep collective wisdom related to dealing with the challenges of life and being human in the ancestral line. They can provide grounding and reassurance in the life process during times of pain and suffering. I will reiterate that this is a relationship building process. It can reflect the type of relationship you would develop with a trusted advisor.

In special cases, where you are certain that there is disruption in your world that is being caused by ancestral patterns, the process of communion can gently be directed towards attempting to shift them. Some patterns may not budge and will require deeper, more nuanced intervention, but sometimes, simple conversations from the heart and offerings can go a long way. In these cases, I would suggest expressing your desire for a particular pattern to shift, and asking for support or for the particular issue to cease. After asking for their help in this, follow it up by giving offerings to make it so and to give thanks. Personally, I would consider this a part of relationship building and communion, rather than ancestral healing, as you're asking for what you need and/or establishing healthy boundaries.

Closing the Conversation

It is often helpful and polite to close the practice somehow. This can be as simple as closing your eyes and intending on it; or you can gently let the spirits know the session is coming to a close and that you appreciated their presence. I sometimes say "Done." a few times to seal the work.

Closing the conversation is good hygiene in my experience.

There you have it. It is that simple to begin your ancestral veneration practice. There are many stages of work, and other layers that this can take on. Although those layers and stages are beyond the scope of this work, I do believe that just about anybody can begin in this way, in a manner that is safe and effective.

CHAPTER 15

May We Plant Seeds of Great Change

"The stars are the campfires of our ancestors."
- Gordon White

Our ancestors are portals into the physical world. They are the doorways through which the endless corridor of the past opens into this plane of existence, allowing us to enter into it. The process of birth and death is a continuous spiraling hallway of creation and destruction; and we are simultaneously walking through it, as well as being a part of it. Consider this through the vantage point of deep time: every life is a fire - a light that burns, smolders, and dies - but before it dies, a small spark ignites yet another flame. Every life in this way is incipient - each life a fractal of the other. And what is more fractal than people literally coming out of other people?

When we talk about ancestors, we also need to talk about karma. In this case, karma being cause and effect, the impact of circumstances and the decisions made within those circumstances; billions of choices feeding into one another and affecting each other. Some might say that fate is just the weight of circumstances. Every moment consists of trillions upon trillions of decisions that weigh upon the possibilities that are present, and act like a massive gravitational pull. Our entrance into this existence is subject to this pull. At a practical level, and beyond the more esoteric avenues this can go, we can say that the time and place we were born determines the culture we find ourselves in, the family and genetics we have, the environment we are exposed to, and the resources we will be able to access during our first few decades. In other words, the ancestral portal - the doorway into this reality - by default, sets each of us up with a fundamental set of causes and conditions or a very large layer of karma.

On a mythological level, stars and destiny have a long history of being interconnected. Many of the world's astrological traditions made this connection despite their diversity. Furthermore, many indigenous traditions also link stars with ancestry. It is believed that the ancestors reside in, or become, the stars when they die, or that the ancestors come from the stars. In addition to these connections, the stars were maps to navigate by, as well as maps to keep track of time, as the old ones understood the stars as keepers of temporal cycles.

The reality of time, choices, cause and effect, and the ancestors reverberating through the ages, underneath a starry sky, illuminates a possibility of why stars, fate, and ancestry are linked throughout the world. If the weight of previous decisions creates the present moment, then this moment could be no other way than what it is. However, this is not static as our decisions are a pulsating web of interactions. Through choice, we begin to shift certain forces and plant our own seeds. We have choice to identify the currents that we are riding, and choice to surf them with more skill. The beautiful truth is, the night sky connects us all. As we stare at the stars, we can take comfort in knowing that for the most part, these are the same stars seen by all of those that came before us. As we look up, we can resonate and can feel back through the fabric of time, contemplating how this makes us one.

I invite you to go out at night to stare at the stars more often. As you do, contemplate the connection you share with the ancestors who also stared at these stars. Feel into the countless decisions that have created a momentum, with one leading to another, leading to you being here now. As you do so, try to understand how the ancestors have been portals through deep time, and opening doorways for the next generation. Try to feel the connection between all of this, and then feel the connection to you, at that moment as you stare up at the stars.

So, what is all of this talk about karma and stars? It is often hindsight that allows us to look back and see the conditions and small developments that lead to great change. At times, we have a limited perception when it comes to any great change, catastrophe, or some sort of windfall - we see them as something that occured suddenly. When huge changes accelerate into being, we often forget that those seeds of change were planted long before the changes came about. With skill and discernment, and after learning to listen, we can start to direct this current of change.

Everyone has a history. Through understanding the impact of that history and integrating what we need, we can then clean the slate. Humanity has been injured and wounded. It is currently trying to stack an advanced civilization on top of a structure that cannot handle it. As a species, we are attempting to shoot a cannon out of a canoe. It's much like the common theme seen with beginners entering into the serious fitness/physical movement cultures. They show up to the new practice with their body exhibiting various dysfunctional compensation patterns that have been set in place over time, and they attempt to stack fitness on top of said dysfunction. The dysfunctional patterns cannot sustain the increased demand being introduced and therefore, it leads to injury. What most beginners in this area need, is taking a step back, improving the patterns of quality, and then focusing on building the horse-power needed after the physical structure has learned that it can handle it. The foundations of our current world cannot sustain the forces being generated as the momentum of human society runs, jumps, and attempts to move around heavy weights. Injury after injury, we continue to move forward and wonder why there is so much trauma and pain in the world. If our abandonment of certain ancestral pathways and the subsequent outcomes that have occurred on a worldwide level are of any indication, then the outcomes of continuing down the current mainstream path do not take much imagination to envision.

The great work of our time is the transmutation of the compensation patterns into healthy, functional patterns. There are many different perspectives on what this entails out there, and Ancestral Now has offered its own take on this work. If we, as individuals and as a species, absorb, integrate, and align with much of our unconscious past, the quality of our movement going forward will be healthier. Small choices can lead to large changes. May we recall that it is through understanding how events, patterns, and trends unfold that we can, at times, predict the future. May the ground substance of our decisions be altered by becoming more whole and integrated homegrown humans. May the seeds that we plant today to improve our lives in the present move through time to impact the future we are all creating together.

www.ingramcontent.com/pod-product-compliance
Lightning Source LLC
Chambersburg PA
CBHW020236130626
46549CB00005B/1915

* 9 7 9 8 2 1 8 0 5 2 6 2 1 *